Metabolic Transformation

Metabolic Transformation

✦

The Ultimate Fat Loss Guide

Dr. Joe Klemczewski

Foreword: Dr. William L. Smith, D.M.D.

iUniverse, Inc.
New York Lincoln Shanghai

Metabolic Transformation
The Ultimate Fat Loss Guide

iUniverse, Inc.

For information address:
iUniverse, Inc.
2021 Pine Lake Road, Suite 100
Lincoln, NE 68512
www.iuniverse.com

Cover Photo: Todd Lucy
Cover Design: Aaron Worthington

ISBN: 0-595-29268-2

Printed in the United States of America

This book is dedicated to my incredibly individual and precious four children, Cameron Joseph, Ashlyn Rebekah, Trey Daniel, and Lynnea Elizabeth. Along with your mother, you are the brightest points in my life. You've seen me dedicate my career to physical medicine and others' health. My hope is that you enjoy lives filled with health, strength, and vitality. Take care of the one body God gave you—you're going to live in it for a long time!

Contents

FOREWORD

I guess in some sort of unacknowledged way, I had given up on myself as far as health and fitness were concerned. After injuries necessitated an end to tennis, my physical activity was confined to the purchase of an expensive machine that was supposed to simulate cross-country skiing. Even in front of the television, skiing was very boring and uncomfortable for my back. Needless to say, the machine was eventually stored away in my attic. I had tried to walk on a regular basis, but I could never sustain for longer than three weeks in a row. It seemed I always had a perfect reason for changing my routine. After all, since I was (very slightly) on the sunny side of 55, I had the rest of my life to "get back in shape."

My diet was miserable, to be honest. When I cut down, it was from a large chocolate bar with almonds to one that weighed one and a half ounces less. My devoted wife of 34 years did her best, but there was no limit to my rationalizing when it came to food consumption.

One day, a good friend of mine that had watched me balloon to approximately 260 pounds left me a semi-subtle hint about a new person in our area that was really good at fitness, nutrition, and motivation. I pretended not to hear him, but later thought of what he had said…most of my waking hours. I had eaten myself off the racks at most clothing stores. Just go to a rack of men's sport coats and see how many 50-long coats there are. Some stores have the nerve to stop at size 48 instead of carrying the one obligatory blue blazer in size 50. I had stopped looking at clothes (except anything that would coordinate with that navy blazer). I had long ago started ordering my shirts from one place that had shirts with 18-inch necks. Most stores stop at 17 and a half, and that was next of kin to a hangman's noose.

After about two weeks of thinking about what my friend had said, I called him and asked for the phone number of this person that could supposedly help me. I was informed that the first step would be a consultation about nutrition. That sounded like something I could handle. I was certainly in good enough condition to sit upright in a chair for 60 minutes, so I made an appointment. When I entered the training facility, I was met by Dr. Joe. He was an attractive, personable, and confident physical specimen that was young enough to be my son. I was not prepared for one of the first questions he asked, "What percentage of body fat do you think you are?" How did this kid have the audacity to ask me such a question?! Did he not know that no one wants to admit that they are half adipose tissue?! By the time the interview was over, I was convinced that he did have some remote grasp of nutrition, even though he had not mentioned chocolate and almonds. I figured I could straighten him out on that later. After six years, I had no luck on this issue. I made an appointment for an hour-long fitness session—more as a comfortable way to end the conversation than as a commitment to a way of life. I could always have my secretary call and cancel (with the message that I would get back to him later). Why should I start something that I knew I would not follow through on? I knew myself well enough…I would rationalize myself out of this in no time.

I guess I waited too long before canceling, so I ended up going out like the proverbial lamb. When I arrived, Dr. Joe told me we were going to do a lower body workout. That was music to my ears because I knew I had a lot of muscle in my legs and he couldn't lay a finger on me. We went to the first machine, which was for my thighs. He placed the pin for the weights under far too light an amount for a man with my legs. At this point, I was hoping I would not damage his machine by pulling the weights though the top; I was sure he had insurance. After less than a three-minute set on this girly-man machine, he informed me that we were moving to another. As I stood up, I thought my legs had been replaced by rubber bands. I got to the next machine by using my hands to steady myself on the other machines (to keep from falling flat on my face). When the hour was over, I was positive that Joe had the "666" mark somewhere under his hair. I would have asked for help to walk to my car, but that would have looked like my final act of submission. In a dazed state, I made another appointment for an upper body workout a couple of days later.

That all started over six years ago. Now, I have regular appointments twice a week. If for some reason I miss two workouts in a row, I start missing it. I feel as though I am wasting away and denying a deep promise I made to myself. I actually feel guilty, a sensation I had never experienced beforehand. I have now lost over 40 pounds of fat and put on several pounds of muscle. I know that some of you will think that after six years of working out, I should have lost more weight. However, when I started this, I promised myself I would lose weight at a rate I could maintain. If I am on vacation and gain a couple pounds, I am not concerned in the least. I do not come home and fast, because I now know that with my present way of life, I will naturally lose the weight. I now weigh 218 pounds and hope to lose another 10 to 20 over the next couple of years. I feel no panic or stress over the outcome of this quest, for I know it will happen.

I have seen Joe make changes in the lives of many people over the last six-plus years. I have seen overweight women transform from introverts in long heavy sweatshirts to model-like figures that cannot posses enough Lycra. Joe connects inwardly with his clients. They know he cares intensely about their progress, and they respond by not wanting to disappoint. It is a deep interpersonal relationship that cannot be explained. He is truly a professional.

Three years ago, I was diagnosed with prostate cancer. One of the first things I did was go to Joe for extra nutritional counseling to prepare my body for the stress of major surgery. He really did not add a whole lot to what I was already doing. I had the surgery on a Monday and was released from the hospital on a Friday. The only real pain I had was when I got up to walk. I was back in my office, essentially working a full schedule, a month after surgery. I had a wonderful surgeon and the blessings and prayers of many. However, I have no doubt, that had I not been in my present condition and living my present lifestyle, my road to recovery would have been much different.

I can also note many ways in which Joe has enhanced my present perspective on life. This goes far beyond the physical me. I now have a more spiritual view of life. Somehow, I have integrated my own body into my spiritual side. My spiritual relationship with my wife has grown much stronger. Joe and I sometimes spend the entire hour of my workout speaking about the spiritual aspects of life. He is totally absorbed in his wife and children. He seems to have every facet of his life together. I have learned much 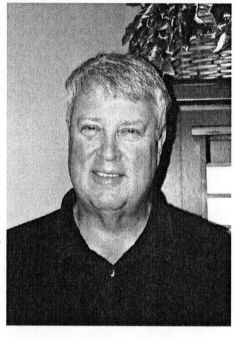 from this man. I can honestly say I am a very different person than I was in June of 1997. I cannot completely define this change, but I know it is there and it is permanent. One of the things in my life that I very much look forward to is the continuation of this change.

These days, I am very thankful for many things in my life…facing cancer was a real eye-opener in terms of where my values should be focused. One thing I am very thankful for is that I have had the opportunity to work with Joe and make this commitment to my life.

When I grow up, I want to be just like Dr. Joe!

William Logan Smith, D.M.D.

PREFACE

This project started four years ago, and every time I sit down to edit or add to it, I feel further away from finishing it. An incurable perfectionist, I would never deem it ready for public view until I've overturned every stone. By limiting myself to one volume, however, I am focusing on exactly what is necessary for success. *Metabolic Transformation* explains complex physiological principles that are critical for permanent weight loss, in a form and style that is easy to understand. Sometimes wisdom supercedes knowledge, and in the case of nutrition and weight loss, they are (at the very least) of equal importance. I have found that a client will rarely succeed without both, and I spend a lot of time devising ways to make weight loss and nutrition easier. This book intertwines physiology and practicality in a concise and—I hope—enlightening way.

As I gained experience helping individual clients reach weight loss and body composition goals, I constantly modified and improved my program's technique and content. Growing public speaking engagements led to the formation of notes, packets, and manuals that eventually funneled into the idea for a book that could be used by my clients and students. The premise was for the book to be fuller in content than my lectures, yet in an easy-to-use format that would increase the likelihood of success. The book itself has also evolved, fueled by my passion to make it a complete work while maintaining its original simplicity.

My formal education has been a natural extension of my fascination with the miraculous complexity of the human body. A bachelor's degree in physical therapy, graduate degrees in health- and nutrition-related fields, and certification as a strength and conditioning specialist are the foundations of my career. However, my own practical nutrition experience as a professional bodybuilder, along with 10 years of nutritional consulting with a broad spectrum of clients, has provided me with the fire to refine my understanding and approach. In its current form, I believe *Metabolic Transformation* exceeds my original intent. This book will certainly become a well-worn reference for those that hear me lecture or are personally involved with my staff and I. However, I also believe it will stand on its own for those that never do more than read it and diligently apply the information herein.

Many will remember the thin manuscript, self-published and spiral-bound. The core text is what has been expanded, and with the help of some good friends, more charts, inserts, and practical application sections have been added. I have also included success stories, personal reflections, and encouragement that is aimed at the joy of living healthily in the amazing one-and-only body that God gives each of us. I also count myself among a demented group of bodybuilders, weight lifters, and fitness enthusiasts that take their bodies to extremes and need cutting-edge nutrition for recovery and performance. Thus, the appendix is a special section of advanced nutrition and aggressive weight-loss techniques.

INTRODUCTION

You've finished college, the "Freshman 15" train has left the station and never come back, and now you find yourself recalling what it was like to look and feel athletic instead of experiencing it. The last of your three children is in school, and you realize you haven't had any time for yourself in over a decade. As you glance in the mirror, you notice you have the physique to prove it. Forty-three years given to your boss, college educations, and the pursuit of the white picket fence, but all your doctor can reward you with is cholesterol meds and the heart attack lecture. Whatever stage of life you find yourself in, I'm glad it has led you to this book. Your physique, your health, and your quality and enjoyment of life hinge on your decision to devote some time to regaining control of your most valuable possession: your body. Consider me your partner, and this book your instruction manual, as we rebuild your temple.

Diet books take up entire sections of bookstores, yet most of us still struggle with our weight. New "experts" emerge almost daily with best-sellers that contain the secrets we've been missing. Despite filling a necessary role in our culture, weight management is an industry with a couple of skeletons rattling in its closet. One fallacy is that if a book is successful, the diet must work. The truth is, most books are successful because those of us that fail on one diet rush out to buy the plan of the next "guru." It's hard to determine the credibility of the author because it's easy to sound like a scientist, and we inherently believe what we read without much discernment. For example, some authors work exclusively with high-level athletes, drug-using bodybuilders, or other narrow populations, and then expect their experiences to carry over to you and me. Or, another trap people fall into is thinking that science is discovering revolutionary new ways of eating with previously undiscovered weight-loss technology. Though perhaps not complete, nutritional science is sound; there is little true controversy in regards to metabolic physiology. In reality, every new diet is a literal repackaging of an old idea dressed up with a great new marketing plan.

So, if new information is minimal and people are getting fatter despite exponential increases in the numbers of experts, books, and diets, why did I write this book? Because I've seen so many diet failures, so much guilt, and so much obsession and misery with lifetime dieting. I've been able to end so much of this misery and help clients return to a superb level of health, functioning, and happiness. I want you to experience the same thing!

In my years of individual nutritional consulting, I haven't run across too many diet novices. My average client has read numerous diet books and has been on many diets yet still struggles. The common thread I've seen over the years has been a fundamental lack of understanding among dieters. Authors are pressured to make their diets easy, so they fill books with recipes, daily menu plans, and detailed instructions for following their diets to the letter. Readers learn how to follow that diet, but they don't learn how to eat or how to maintain their weight. In short, they don't learn what it takes to function in a society with little spare time, too much fast food, and temptation galore. My clients succeed when they learn how to become their own nutritionists, which is my goal for them. This is also my goal for you.

Nutrition isn't just about science; it also takes practicality. You can be holding steady on the perfect diet and yet fail at managing nutrition in the real world. I studied nutrition formally for years, stay current with research, and read journals and new text books constantly, but that knowledge is only part of what has given my clients success. I have learned much of what I know about weight loss because I must diet to a ridiculously low level of body fat for professional body-building contests. I've also learned from the real world experiences of my clients. I, by the way, am among the world's worst dieters. I am a borderline endomorph stuck with a moderately high "metabolic set point" for body fat storage and I don't have the greatest level of discipline when it comes to food—I love to eat! My own dieting and weight management have given me practical experience that often leads to insight and the development of new methods for easier "survival" while losing body fat. I also have learned immensely from every client that brings unique circumstances to the same battle. I work with world champion body-builders, homemakers, and everyone in between.

As with most areas in life, you just can't place nice borders around the topic of weight loss and how your body looks. It's a topic that oozes over boundaries that you think are firmly in place. What I mean is that some assume that their body fat level is genetically determined, period. Others think it's all mental discipline. Still more say that there are laws of physiology in play that make eating one way better than another. Guess what? They're all right. I will convince you that dieting and your physique is limited by genetics, but not defined by them. I will show you that there are certain physiological rules to nutrition that make it easier to lose weight and keep it off. I'll also probably disappoint you by saying that even though it's easier when you "do things right," it also takes some discipline at times. I mean, hey, a cheeseburger is always going to taste better than tuna!

Through the journey of physiology, practicality, and new knowledge, I also want to help some readers overcome guilt, shame, and obsession over appearance. Obesity is looked down upon as gluttony and a product of laziness and zero self-discipline. But let me remind you that there is a proven genetic component of body structure and body fat storage tendencies. It is much harder for some people to lose weight than others, and it's much easier for these people to gain weight. That isn't a life-sentence for being overweight, for anyone can make the choice to eat properly, but it's still very difficult physically for some people. For those that would point a scornful finger at the belt-line of another, could it be that there are imperfections that aren't so easy to see hidden behind the sunken cheeks of another? My point is that your success in weight loss will undoubtedly lead to self-confidence but your self-worth shouldn't be found in your body fat percentage. I hope you're just as concerned with what's on the inside, so let's make quick work of taking care of the outside!

Don't let me throw the baby out with the bath water, however. We obsess about our appearances while 25,000 people a day die of starvation around the world. Do you catch my drift? Let's learn how to eat properly for the best health and best function of our bodies; a side effect, of course, is that we look and feel better, but let's not obsess about it. Let's get on with the more important joys that God created us for!

Metabolic Transformation will help you become your own nutritionist and free you to spend your life on greater pursuits as a happier and healthier person. It's a book that's scientifically pointed but also peppered with tips, ideas, and strategies that will help you win the war for control. Now, let's head for the front lines!

1

METABOLISM: TURNING YOUR BODY INTO A FAT-BURNING MACHINE

Metabolism Defined

Not long ago, a 44-year-old man came to me with a goal of getting leaner and possibly gaining some muscle. He already enjoyed a lifestyle of working out and running almost every day, and had done so for most of his adult life. Despite being very healthy from this physical training perspective, he gained and lost 20 pounds more than once and lamented his lack of control. He wanted to lose weight again, but he also wanted a permanent revolution and permanent control. This of course, forces thoughts of success as a mental obstacle. Perhaps my client needed a master motivator to drive his consciousness up to a higher level of passion regarding his abs and biceps. Perhaps I could hypnotize him and plant subconscious links between Twinkies and rat poison. Without fail, I've found the greatest link to success, however, is to help people get their metabolic physiology in order and, in the process, teach them how and why we're doing it. Nutritional knowledge brings about physical changes, becomes internalized by positive reinforcement (seeing the changes), and can only be fully implemented at will after this mixture of knowledge and self-experience is realized.

My new client lost 20 pounds of body fat and gained five pounds of lean body mass in his first eight weeks. How can a man that already exercises regularly, works out with weights at least four days per week, and runs in road races have such dramatic results just by changing his nutrition? The answer is metabolism. He actually complained about having to eat so much food on his program, and after those first eight weeks, I had to increase his food so he wouldn't lose weight "too quickly." He often commented on his new, higher level of energy. A very disciplined, in-control person, he went as far to say, "Coming to you literally changed my life." Are these comments typical with dieters you know? Not hardly! Study after study has shown that most dieters regain even more weight than they lose on any given plan.

How many times have you heard people say they have a fast or slow metabolism? Thin people often say, "I have a fast metabolism," and those who are overweight often say, "I have a slow metabolism." We are quick to blame or credit our body size on a word that most of us don't even understand. Basal metabolic rate is the rate at which your body burns calories over a specific amount of time. It's true that there is some variability in everyone's metabolism; however, I have met few people who had a legitimately "slow" metabolism due to a thyroid imbalance, metabolic condition, or medical ailment that would compromise weight loss. In other words, your metabolism may be slightly lower than someone else's, but it's probably not the reason you are overweight.

An analogy is blaming breast cancer on genetics. True, there is a gene mutation that causes breast cancer. If a woman has this gene, she will get breast cancer, but this gene causes only 10 percent of breast cancer cases. The other 90 percent are brought about by other causes. In that same light, the cause of your weight struggle likely goes beyond your genetic metabolism.

Don't misunderstand me. While I'm downplaying the role of metabolism as an excuse, it does play a great role in major long-term impact in the bigger picture of weight management. What you eat does affect your metabolism. Within weeks, you can raise or lower your body's ability to burn calories, sometimes significantly. Over time, this change can add up to large weight loss or gain. To be quite honest, this is the foundation of permanent weight loss. By eating the right amount of food, eating within the right daily structure, consuming better ratios of the three macronutrients (protein, carbohydrates, and fat), selecting the right food choices, and learning to be consistent, you can actually increase the amount of calories your body burns per day. This change in metabolism is due to the optimum operation of your body's internal environment.

(Figure 1:1) Basal Metabolic Rate:

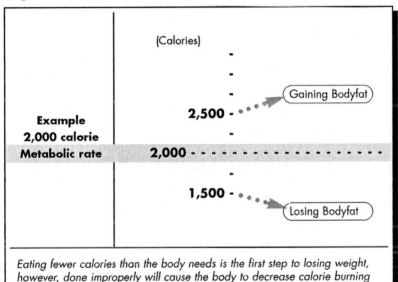

Eating fewer calories than the body needs is the first step to losing weight, however, done improperly will cause the body to decrease calorie burning making it easier to gain body fat. Permanent positive changes in metabolism will occur only through the combined results of eating nutrients in the right amounts in a structured meal plan.

When you diet or eat incorrectly, your body does not work at optimum levels. Know anyone that has lost 30 pounds only to gain 40 back? They may insist they didn't gorge themselves to regain the weight, but simply started eating "normally." Incorrect dieting can reduce the amount of calories your body burns, therefore making it much easier to gain weight even though you're trying to lose weight.

Pay close attention to the details of this book as we explore how your body works with correct nutrition.

Eating the Right Amount to Raise Your Metabolism

As we progress through specific nutrient information and physiology, you will clearly see how the amount, type, and consumption pattern of food can literally accelerate your metabolism to full throttle. The first and most important step, however, is to estimate your metabolic rate correctly so you can eat the amount of food that allows you to reach your weight loss goals. Once you know how much energy your body requires, you can adjust your eating downward to begin the weight loss process.

You could logically assume that eating five calories less than your body requires burns five extra calories stored as body fat, or that if you consume 500 calories less, your body makes up the difference by burning 500 calories of stored fat. Actually, the process is more complex than this. There is far more to permanent weight loss than just reducing calories. For instance, the body can burn calories by catabolizing, or breaking down, other tissues, such as muscle. Other "intermediate" sources of energy such as blood sugar and stored carbohydrates (glycogen) in the liver and muscle may be used as well. Thus, the goal is to maximize fat loss while sparing muscle. There is a fine line between losing the most body fat as fast as possible and doing it in such a way that your metabolism is raised and not lowered.

The first step, therefore, is to determine the amount of food necessary to reach your goal. I have developed a chart based on gender and height to make this most important step very easy. This chart ensures enough food to avoid any deficiencies in the three macronutrients, is geared towards a one-to-two pound weight loss per week, and encompasses the entire material content in this book. A great deal of experience and human trial has been poured into this chart to make it the simplest yet most powerful tool you have ever had in your battle for permanent weight control. It seems too easy to just plug yourself into a chart and follow the numbers, but therein lies the challenge. It will require discipline to stay with your program. Most people reading this will not have a clear concept regarding the numbers on the chart. In other words, most cannot correlate how much food is required to eat 100 grams of protein, or even which foods contain protein. Fear not: within six weeks, you will be on the way to becoming your own nutritionist.

What if it Doesn't Seem to be Working?

Everything we will explore from this point on will expand this one simple step of consuming the right amounts of the right macronutrients. I will expand and explain a great deal of information that will make this step even easier, yet it remains your responsibility to stay within your suggested total ranges.

We have established that everyone is different metabolically, and therefore, this chart may not be a perfect fit for some readers. The goal is to lose one-to-two pounds of body fat per week, and this chart was created for the general population with a moderate activity level. You may lose five-to-seven pounds the first week due to water loss, but one-to-two pounds each week thereafter is the goal. If, despite following your totals perfectly, eating the best food selections as described, and using the methods in this book, you are not obtaining the desired results, you may need to make an adjustment. First, if you are not losing weight fast enough (one-to-two pounds per week), make sure you're eating at the low end of the chart ranges. If you are losing too rapidly, make sure you're eating at the high end of the chart ranges. If you're still losing too fast, add 25 grams of carbohydrates to your daily totals for a week and reassess your results. Keep adding until you are losing at the desired one-to-two pound-per-week rate. If you are still losing too slowly (even at the low end of your suggested chart totals), drop your daily intake of carbs by 10 grams for a week and reassess. If necessary, repeat this until you are losing weight at the appropriate rate.

(Figure 1:2) Food Volume Chart

Height		Men:	Women:
		(Grams per day)	
5' - 5'4"			
	Protein	120 - 140	70 - 90
	Carbohydrates	140 - 170	90 - 120
	Fat	45 - 55	25 - 30
	(Calories)	(1,445 - 1,735)	(865 - 1,110)
5'5" - 5'8"			
	Protein	140 - 160	80 - 100
	Carbohydrates	160 - 190	100 - 130
	Fat	50 - 60	30 - 35
	(Calories)	(1,650 - 1,940)	(990 - 1,235)
5'9" - 6'			
	Protein	160 - 180	90 - 110
	Carbohydrates	180 - 210	110 - 140
	Fat	55 - 65	35 - 40
	(Calories)	(1,855 - 2,145)	(1,115 - 1,360)
6'1" - 6'4"			
	Protein	180 - 200	100 - 120
	Carbohydrates	200 - 230	120 - 150
	Fat	60 - 70	40 - 45
	(Calories)	(2,060 - 2,350)	(1,240 - 1,485)
6'5" - 6'8"			
	Protein	200 - 220	110 - 130
	Carbohydrates	220 - 250	130 - 160
	Fat	65 - 75	45 - 50
	(Calories)	(2,265 - 2,555)	(1,365 - 1,610)

Metabolic Transformation in Action

"Like countless other Americans, I too was delusional thinking that my slim, lean, 98 pound physique would remain so regardless of the excessive consumption of fatty, sugary, high-calorie foods. During my high school years, I was the girl who could eat anything and not gain weight. On many occasions I had no second thoughts about eating a large pizza and a half-gallon of ice cream in a single sitting. Needless to say, I was the envy of all my friends!

Equipped with no adequate nutritional insight I dragged my excessive eating patterns into college. As a result, a sophomore, junior, and senior fifteen followed the "freshman fifteen". Each year I became more and more devastated by my weight gains and I became more and more determined to take control of my weight. Consequently, I tried a myriad of diets and weight loss programs, to no avail. My futile attempts to shed my excess weight resulted in a shocking 150-pound weight upon graduation.

Returning home after graduation was a very stressful time for me, as I knew my family and friends would clearly note, and secretly comment, on my hefty weight gain. The embarrassment quickly prompted me to join the local gym and begin attending group exercise classes. Unfortunately for me, it was not enough. The weight wasn't coming off. In an ardent attempt to find a sure-fire solution, I began to read more in an effort to educate myself on successful strategies for weight loss. I discovered that I not only needed a cardio component in my fitness regime, I needed weight training as well. Soon I was pushing iron, running, doing step aerobics, and kickboxing. A barrage of compliments by friends and family rewarded my hard work.

My enthusiasm for fitness led me to seek and procure certification as a fitness instructor and personal trainer. Although I had attained a level of fitness and status many were awed by, a voided question of continued success remained. I would begin to fill that void by attending my first bodybuilding show. I recall being surrounded by people from an elite fitness class and dreaming of a day when I would grace the stage with a fit, lean, muscular physique. At that moment, I decided to make my dream a reality.

I now had a relatively decent level of general nutritional knowledge, but I needed something more in-depth. Through inquiries, I was introduced to Nancy Andrews, two-time WNBF World Bodybuilding Champion, who encouraged me to attend her Pro Series Bodybuilding Camp. From the onset, I gained a wealth of new knowledge that still amazes me today.

continued ⟶

Metabolic Transformation in Action

While attending the weekend workshop, I was introduced to the "Guru of Nutrition," Dr. Joe Klemczewski. Dr. Joe's expertise on weight loss was impressive not only because of his extensive knowledge, but because he was able to articulate it in a manner that was easy to comprehend. Through his support and guidance, I was finally able to understand how to retain my weight loss and even take my physique to a new level.

When I did enter my first ever figure and bodybuilding competition, I placed an unbelievable first and second place respectively. I continue to work with Dr. Joe via email, making adjustments to my nutrition as my goals change. His unabated support, expertise, and encouragement brought me from a vision of merely walking across a stage to standing on that stage as a two-time winner! Thanks, Joe!"

Enieda, Probation Officer and Fitness Instructor

What To Expect The First Week

As briefly mentioned, your body has many sources of energy to draw from. When anyone lowers calorie intake below what is necessary (basal metabolic rate), the caloric deficit must be made up from somewhere. Though we would all like it to be body fat that is used, there is actually a percentage of energy taken from almost every available source. The most readily available is blood sugar, and then liver glycogen (stored sugar). These are dynamic, easy-to-access energy stores that are immediately used when needed. Muscle glycogen is a large area of stored energy, but its primary purpose is for muscle contraction and work, and it is therefore not as easily retrieved for maintenance calorie needs. Between meals, body fat is released from body fat cells, but only as much is as needed. So, if you follow the path, this paragraph will be monumental to your understanding. Your food intake must be precise and consistent so that you will get precise and consistent results. The total amount of calories is moderately lower than what your body needs on a daily basis, therefore it needs a secondary source of calories. The first things your body is going to access are blood sugar, liver glycogen, and a moderate amount of available muscle glycogen (especially if you work out). The food intake chart is designed to take a large portion of the caloric deficit from carbohydrates so that as you continue using blood sugar and glycogen, you will eventually (within 2-4 days) be as depleted as your brain will safely allow. Blood sugar levels are critical to the brain and body, so your brain won't let you go too far without throwing a tantrum. At this point, you'll feel hungry, possibly weak and shaky, maybe tired, and some will even get a headache. You now have reached a level of carbohydrate depletion that opens a door to significant body fat loss. If you give in to the hunger at this point, you'll refill your muscle and liver glycogen as well as your blood stream glucose (sugar), and you'll have to start over. Unfortunately, this is a pattern of many dieters. Three or four days go well and then a binge sends them back to the starting point, both physically and mentally. What happens in reality is that they deplete and replete carb stores without much alteration in body fat, and though they really are eating well 80 percent of the time, they don't lose weight.

If, however, you stay within your suggested food total ranges through this "tough" day of being carb-depleted, a great advancement takes place. Since you're not giving in to the carb cravings, your brain is forced into plan B. Plan B is that since you're not providing more glucose (sugar) from your diet, your body has to find another source. I can't emphasize enough how amazing the design of our bodies is. Two things will now happen that allow for immediate and consistent body fat loss. Body fat cells start releasing fatty acids and glycerol, the products of stored body fat. Once in the bloodstream, some is used directly by certain types of cells for energy, and some actually gets converted into glucose. This mechanism, called "gluconeogenesis," is literally the creation of new glucose from non-carbohydrate sources, which can be fat or protein. Now, blood sugar levels come back up to a consistent level so energy returns and hunger decreases. As a matter of fact, there is almost a euphoric rise in energy and a marked decrease in lethargy throughout the day due to the consistency in blood sugar. As long as you're consistent with your suggested food intake totals, you're now making up the majority of the caloric deficit through the mechanism of turning your body fat into new carbohydrates. We can survive for long periods of time by accessing these stored calories in the form of body fat, if necessary. Understanding how to safely and effectively take advantage of this design is how you're going to lose body fat permanently and without the torment of fad diets.

One note is that each gram of glycogen holds approximately three times its weight in water. A by-product of cellular metabolism is also water. So, the first week of decreasing your body's level of stored carbohydrates and beginning the process of losing body fat will result in a large amount of water loss. It isn't uncommon for someone to lose five to eight pounds in the first week. The second week's weight loss will be a truer reflection of how much body fat is being lost.

Exercise and Metabolism

One note about exercise: exercise increases caloric output. You can (and should) accelerate body fat loss through a structured workout regimen. After your physician has decreed that it is safe for you to work out, choose a type of exercise program that you can enjoy and continue. If you're interested in maximum results, losing the most body fat, and building the most muscle, contact the best personal trainer you can find.

(Figure 1:3) Sample Food Count Chart

	Protein	Carbs	Fat
High Protein Foods			
Chicken Breast (4 oz)	28	0	4
Chicken Thigh (4 oz)	20	0	8
Turkey Breast (4 oz)	28	0	4
Fish (4 oz)	26	0	1
Ground Beef (4 oz	27	0	24
Ground Beef, Lean (4 oz)	29	0	19
Flank Steak (4 oz)	30	0	14
Egg White	4	0	0
Egg Yolk	3	0	5
(All measurements in cooked form)			
High Carbohydrate Foods:			
Oats (1/2 cup dry)	5	27	3
Baked Potato (1 cup)	3	26	1
Baked Sweet Potato (1 cup)	2	38	0
White Rice (1/4 cup dry)	4	35	1
Brown Rice (1/4 cup dry)	4	34	1
Whole Wheat Bread (1 sl.)	3	12	1
Broccoli (1 cup)	1	5	0
Green Beans (1 cup)	2	8	0
Lettuce (1 cup)	1	2	0
Carrots (1 cup)	1	11	0
Corn (1 cup)	5	42	2
Pasta (1 cup cooked)	7	40	1
Apple (3" diameter)	1	24	0
Banana (5 oz)	1	33	0
High Fat Foods:			
Olive Oil (1 Tbsp.)	0	0	14
Flaxseed Oil (1 Tbsp.)	0	0	11
Peanut Butter (1 Tbsp.)	5	4	8
Almonds (1/4 cup)	5	5	15

(Corinne T. Netzer's book, The Complete Book of Food Counts, is highly recommended to assist in tracking your food intake.)

CHAPTER ONE KEY POINTS

» » » »»► 1) Correct nutrition can raise your metabolism to help achieve
weight loss.

» » » »»► 2) The right amount of food per day is the first and most important
step in achieving permanent and predictable weight loss through
raising your metabolism.

» » » »»► 3) You must follow your macronutrient totals consistently to achieve
this predictable body fat loss. (These will be further defined in
later chapters.)

» » » »»► 4) It may be necessary to adjust your macronutrient totals.

» » » »»► 5) After two to four days, be prepared to feel hungry, tired,
and possibly get a headache as your body prepares to begin
converting body fat into glucose. Stay on course, it will only last
one day at the most.

» » » »»► 6) Be patient with the amount of information you are learning.
It will continue to make more sense as you continue reading.

2

MEAL STRUCTURING

Meal Portions

Now that you have established how much food you need per day, how are you to structure this food into your daily meals and snacks? This question is far more important than you might think. You can actually gain or lose weight eating the exact same amount of food just by changing how you schedule your meals during the day.

There is a limit to how much food your body can effectively digest, metabolize, and absorb at one time. If you eat too much at a meal, some of that food ends up stored as new body fat. So even if you're eating the right amount of food per day, you could be working against yourself by storing new body fat at certain meals. At best, this could slow your progress; at worst, it could negate any progress at all. This pattern can result from our culture's typical way of eating: skip breakfast, grab a candy bar or burger at lunch, and then start supper in the kitchen and extend until bedtime via a well-worn track from the couch to the refrigerator. Not only does this style of eating promote consuming too much at one time, it also means going for long periods of time without eating. This brings up another problem.

Once digestion, absorption, and metabolism have slowed and stopped after a meal, your body starts using stored energy. If you go too long without eating, your metabolic processes slow down to conserve energy. So, if you eat only a couple of large meals per day, your body starts converting the excess food from large meals into body fat. During the long spaces between meals, your metabolism slows down. Essentially, you have created a downward spiral of storing new body fat, and then making it easier to store even more due to a slowing metabolism.

Power Spacing

It is also important to eat small meals and snacks more frequently, totaling five to seven a day. By frequently eating meals small enough so they are completely absorbed and not stored as body fat, you can keep your metabolism charged to maximal levels.

Several factors can make it easy to design your meal spacing plan. First and foremost, divide the quantity of macronutrients logically, not necessarily perfectly, but logically. Two-to-three meals per day should be solid; normal meals, much the same as you may currently eat, except in the right amounts. (Food choices and actual meals with macronutrient ratios will be discussed in later chapters.) The remaining two-to-three meals per day will be smaller snacks. Try to eat your meals or snacks every three-to-four hours.

(Figure 2:1) Sample Meal Plan

6:00 a.m.	Breakfast
9:00 a.m.	Snack
12:00 p.m.	Lunch
3:00 p.m.	Snack
6:00 p.m.	Supper
9:00 p.m.	Small snack (optional)

Having provided an overview of the importance of meal spacing, I want you to know exactly why this step is so important. Recall from Chapter One that your body is essentially in a constant stage of metabolic storage or retrieval. Blood nutrient levels are being kept steady by the constant work of virtually every system of your body. After a meal, the body is working to digest and distribute nutrients in a pattern based on priority. Seemingly frantic processes are occurring to keep the body functioning at its highest level. As those critical process needs are being met, however, excess food is quickly stored, since it is not needed at that particular time. Remember, the body is built for survival. What it doesn't need now, it will store to use later. Excess fat in a meal can be stored directly as fat right out of the bloodstream, and excess carbohydrates will be converted into fat. Both of these processes will be discussed in depth in later chapters.

The bottom line is that too much food in one meal will create new body fat on the premise that your body will be able to use it later. Even with people whose weight is very stable, this happens constantly. We store a little body fat and then use it between meals. Those of us that carry more weight than is healthy, though, are walking reminders that we're storing more at those meals than we're ultimately using. The answer isn't to wait longer between meals, it's to not overeat at meals and stop the process before it starts. This is critically important because we store body fat so much more easily than we use it. Once digestion and absorption are complete after a meal, and our blood sugar levels start to lower, we now have to work our way through the newly stored glycogen in the liver and the blood lipids (fat) before we start using a larger portion of stored body fat. Sometimes we may never even get to that level before we eat again and restart the process.

Conversely, if we eat meals that contain "just the right amount" of protein, carbohydrates, and fat to allow our body to function optimally, we increase the likelihood of not storing anything new as fat, and then spend more time between meals in a retrieval mode, burning stored body fat for energy. You'll find that you're ready for that next meal even if you're not used to eating frequently. You can quickly create a pattern of stability in your metabolism that keeps blood nutrient levels from fluctuating wildly, energy levels high, and body fat usage constant. The alternative of eating larger, less frequent meals will lead to slower weight loss, potential weight gain, and fatigue.

Metabolic Transformation in Action

"At forty-five years old, I learned that anything is possible when you are determined, disciplined, and willing to sacrifice to reach your goal. In July 2000, I was unhappy and disappointed with how life had turned out. I weighed 172 pounds and was on the verge of a size sixteen. I made a twenty-dollar bet with a co-worker to see who could lose the most weight in an eight-week period. I lost seventeen pounds and won the bet.

I signed up at a gym to include exercise in my program and after an orientation with the owner, I could barely move for several days! I didn't get discouraged and soon I became what seemed like a permanent fixture in the gym. Not long after that, my hard work started paying off. I started receiving compliments on my appearance, which fueled my determination to be the best I could.

I even entered a figure competition. Even though I didn't win, I didn't get discouraged. I met Art Archer at the show, who was speaking at a seminar, and he signed a photo, "Joycie, Have faith and stay focused!" That turned out to be the best advice I had ever gotten.

That led to me consulting with Dr. Joe to really get nutrition under my belt. Nutrition has been the most important factor in my weight loss. By eating five to six small meals a day I found that I never over ate and my energy stayed up. Three meals consisted of food while the other three were mainly made up of protein drinks or bars. My diet consisted of baked chicken, fish, turkey and steamed vegetables with lots of water to drink. I also allowed myself one cheat meal a week as part of the plan Joe created for me. Keeping a food logbook helped me keep close tabs on my intake of protein, carbs and fat grams. I also found that weighing my food with a food scale to the exact portions made it easy for me.

Working with Joe and training hard, my muscles exploded and my confidence soared! I was more determined and focused than ever before. By October 2002, I was the leanest I had ever been in my life. I started receiving compliments everywhere I went!

I've learned a lot about myself and a lot about life. I started with a goal and it evolved through the positive changes. The goal inspired and motivated my to move onto new goals. In fact, I have just started studying to become a certified personal trainer.

continued ⟶

Metabolic Transformation in Action

It all begins with you. Make sure you're doing it for you and no one else. Keep an upbeat attitude and stay focused and motivated. Take time out to re-evaluate your goals and make changes accordingly. Try to overcome your setbacks no matter how defeating they look. I'm forty-five years old; it's never too late to succeed. If I can do it, so can you! You CAN accomplish your goals!"

Joycie, Administrative Assistant

The Convenience Factor

Eating five to seven times a day poses a scheduling challenge to most people. However, once you have adopted this new way of eating, you will have so much more energy that you'll never want to revert to your past meal pattern. Eating small, frequent meals keeps nutrients flowing into your body, which is the cornerstone of good health and weight management. Blood sugar, nitrogen (protein), and blood lipid levels all stay more uniform via small meals. Everyone has experienced lulls (and even crashes) in energy during the day. With well-spaced meals, these lulls will disappear and be replaced with steady, high energy levels.

You can easily overcome meal-scheduling challenges with good planning. Meal replacement drinks ("protein shakes") and high-quality food bars can be very good, convenient snack choices. Low-glycemic fruit (as discussed in Chapter 3), yogurt, and many other whole-food choices are also easy to fit into your daily routine. The point is, you have to plan ahead to make sure you can eat when you should eat.

CHAPTER TWO KEY POINTS

• • • •▶ 1) Too much food at one meal leads to new body fat storage.

• • • •▶ 2) Too much time between meals slows the metabolism.

• • • •▶ 3) Five to seven small meals/snacks can maximize metabolic rate and keep body fat loss consistent.

• • • •▶ 4) Well-planned and spaced meals will lead to steady, high energy levels throughout the entire day.

• • • •▶ 5) Convenience is very important. Plan ahead to make sure you can eat when you should.

3

CARBOHYDRATES

Friend or Foe?

Chapters One and Two answered structural questions: How much should I eat and how should I create and space my meals? Now the discussion moves directly to food. Food is divided into three main macronutrients: protein, carbohydrates, and fat. Each is dramatically different both in structure and function. A calorie isn't just a calorie. Each macronutrient will be covered in its own chapter. We begin with the most controversial.

Many dietitians and nutritionists have elevated carbohydrates to an almost untouchable level of nutritional deity. For decades, "experts" have devised weight loss schemes with carbohydrates at the center of the diets. Commercials still brag about how cereals are full of "nutritious carbohydrates."

Long before nutrition was a studied science, it was understood that athletes needed more fuel—more calories—to support their training. Then, like now, carbohydrates were the most abundant, least expensive, most convenient, and (for the most part) best-tasting food. Since athletes were observed consuming many more carbohydrates than anyone else and had physiques that were admired by all, the conclusion was drawn that eating carbs was the way to go. My more science-oriented readers may already be able to conclude that correlation does not equal causation. Athletes may be able to eat a great deal of carbohydrates and not gain body fat due to their intense levels of training, but what about those of us that don't train as hard? And just because athletes may "get away" with eating too many carbs because of their energy expenditure, does that mean it's the best nutrition? Even for them?

Of course, the answer to one extreme is always the opposite extreme, so it didn't take long for no-carbohydrate diets to slither onto the scene. To answer these questions and cut our way through a still raging controversy, let's turn to metabolic physiology. Once you understand exactly what happens inside your body when you eat different foods, you'll be able to discern good nutrition from bad.

(Figure 3:1) Carbohydrate Digestion

Stomach

Digestion occurs in the stomach. The amount of time required partly depends on the complexity of the carb source.

Intestine

Absoprtion occurs in the small intestine once the carbs have been converted to glucose.

Carbohydrate Structure and Function

Carbohydrates provide most of the energy for our bodies most of the time. Because they require the least energy to digest, carbohydrates are the easiest of the macronutrients to digest and be converted to glucose, or blood sugar. Carb sources are loosely described as sugars, starches, or fibers, and these are commonly described as simple and complex carbo-hydrates. We typically think of simple carbohydrates as junk food, like soda and candy, and complex carbs as whole foods, like potatoes, pasta, and bread. This type of categorization leads to the false assumption that a particular food is either good or bad when actually, there is more of a continuum that allows a more detailed comparison. Good, better, best, bad, and/or worse may be more appropriate ways of describing carb choices once you understand how they compare to one another and how they affect your body.

Glucose is the smallest sugar molecule possible. It is the form of sugar that the human body uses for energy. Whatever form of carbohydrate you consume, the end result of digestion is glucose. There are, however, many forms of carbohydrates, and the pathway of digestion that leads to glucose is what can affect our energy levels, mental acuity, physical functioning, and even athletic performance.

You may recognize the names of various forms of sugar: glucose, lactose, fructose, maltose, dextrose, sucrose, and so on. Each one of these carbohydrates has a different level of molecular complexity. Those that are made primarily of glucose are easy and quick to digest since most of the carbs are already in the smallest possible form. Those with a more complex molecular structure are harder to digest and take longer to move through the digestion process. The *Glycemic Index* (Fig. 3:6) is a scale that ranks carbohydrate foods by comparing their structures. It reveals the simplicity or complexity of the sugar, starch, and fiber that make up the macronutrient called carbohydrates.

When you consume a high-glycemic index carbohydrate such as white bread, a banana, a baked potato, soda, candy, etc., you are consuming a carbohydrate that is primarily glucose, the smallest sugar molecule possible. Since glucose is the form of sugar that our bodies use for energy, little digestion needs to take place with these foods. They pass through the stomach quickly and enter the small intestine. Absorption occurs in the small intestine, and since so much glucose enters so fast, sugar uptake is rapid. Your brain closely monitors your blood sugar levels, and such a rapid increase triggers your pancreas to release the hormone insulin. Insulin is a storage hormone that shuttles blood glucose where it is needed.

(Figure 3:2) Insulin Reaction

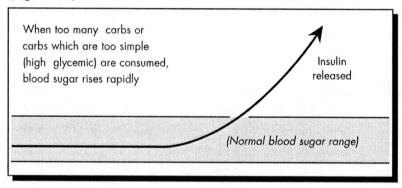

Most of us aren't glycogen-depleted (short of stored glucose), and our muscles and livers usually contain plenty of glucose. So, depending on how many carbohydrates you consume at one time, chances are you will still have too much blood glucose and nowhere to store it. Insulin is still present in high amounts with the elevated levels of glucose, and this causes your liver to convert the blood glucose into triglycerides (fat) to be ultimately stored.

(Figure 3:3) Carbohydrate Conversion to Body Fat

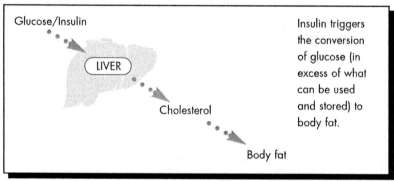

None of the aforementioned high-glycemic carb sources have fat in them, but a large portion of the carbs can be converted to body fat due to insulin sensitivity, as described in the previous paragraph. Unfortunately, the problems don't stop there. Once insulin drops, be it by storage or by fat conversion, your blood glucose levels return to normal, and your brain tells your pancreas to stop releasing insulin. However, even with the process stopped, a certain amount of insulin remains active in the bloodstream until it is "used up." This means more blood sugar will be removed, dropping it below the normal level. A blood sugar level that's too low will leave you tired and possibly weak and shaky. Even worse, your brain sends out powerful hormonal messengers to signal hunger. Have you ever ended up weak, shaky, and starving just 30 or 60 minutes after eating?

(Figure 3:4) Insulin Overcompensation

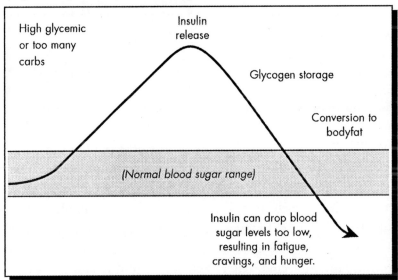

High glycemic or too many carbs

Insulin release

Glycogen storage

Conversion to bodyfat

(Normal blood sugar range)

Insulin can drop blood sugar levels too low, resulting in fatigue, cravings, and hunger.

The tragedy of this whole process is it takes you from bad to worse in body composition, energy levels, and health in one fell swoop. You either block body fat loss or store new body fat with a "fat free" food, you end up tired, and then you're so hungry with carbohydrate cravings that you eat a similar meal and start the process all over again.

This is an extremely powerful bio-chemical reaction. Massive, seemingly uncontrollable binges are birthed by insulin-induced low blood sugar. Many of us live on this roller coaster and don't realize that we're the ones causing it. "I just have a slow metabolism" or "You just naturally gain more body fat as you get older"—I know you've used these excuses, and I know you've believed them. It's time to gain control over your nutrition for good!

(Figure 3:5) Stable Blood Sugar Through Carbohydrate Management

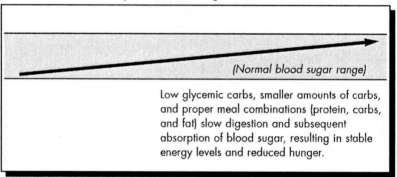

(Normal blood sugar range)

Low glycemic carbs, smaller amounts of carbs, and proper meal combinations (protein, carbs, and fat) slow digestion and subsequent absorption of blood sugar, resulting in stable energy levels and reduced hunger.

What if you chose a carbohydrate on the other end of the glycemic index, such as a grapefruit, an apple, a bowl of oatmeal, or even a salad? These carb sources have different molecular configurations of glucose. Fructose, cellulose, galactose, etc., are much more complex forms of carbohydrate. When these hit your stomach, digestion takes longer to break them into usable glucose molecules. Since this process takes more time, the molecules enter the small intestine and are absorbed more gradually. Blood sugar levels now rise more slowly, avoiding a major insulin reaction. Just by changing the carb source, you have decreased the potential for the creation of new body fat, and your energy level rises over the next couple of hours instead of plummeting quickly. Possibly best of all for someone that is dieting, your hunger is dramatically reduced because your blood glucose levels are stable instead of too low, such as at the end of an insulin rampage.

(Figure 3:6) Sample Glycemic Index Selections

The glycemic index essentially rates the speed of digestion of carbohydrates and thus the impact on blood sugar elevation. A zero rating could indicate no carbohydrates present, glucose is rated at a value of 100, and very simple carbohydrates can reach a value much higher than 100.

	Glycemic Index Value	Serving Size	Grams of Carbs per Serving
CEREALS AND BREADS			
All Bran®	30	1/2 cup	15
Bran Flakes™	74	1/2 cup	18
Corn Flakes™	92	1 cup	26
Crispix™	87	1 cup	25
Grape Nuts™	75	1/4 cup	22
Raisin Bran™	61	1/2 cup	19
Rice Krispies™	87	1 cup	21
Oatmeal (rolled oats)	42	1/2 cup (dry)	27
Shredded Wheat™	75	1 cup	30
Special K™	69	1 cup	21
Bagel, white	72	1	70
English Muffin	77	1	14
Oatbran bread	47	1	18
Pancakes	67	2-4"	58
Rye bread	58	1 slice	14
Whole wheat bread	77	1 slice	12
White bread	80	1 slice	14
SNACKS			
Blueberry muffin	59	3.5 oz	47
Ironman PR Bar®	39	2.3 oz	26
METRx Bar®	74	3.6 oz	50
Pretzels	83	1 oz	20
Potato chips	57	2 oz	18
Soda crackers	74	5	15
Rice cake	82	1	7
Tortilla chips	63	2 oz	30

	Glycemic Index Value	Serving Size	Grams of Carbs per Serving
COMMON "STARCH" SOURCES FOR MEALS			
Instant white rice	87	1/2 cup	28
Potato, baked	85	5 oz	30
Rice, brown	50	1/2 cup	17
Rice, long grain	61	1/2 cup	18
Pasta, white	38	1 cup	32
Pasta, wheat	32	1 cup	32
Sweet potato	44	5 oz	25
FRUIT			
Apple	38	4 oz	15
Banana	52	4 oz	24
Cantaloupe	65	4 oz	6
Cherries	22	1/2 cup	10
Grapefruit	25	1/2	11
Grapes	46	1 cup	24
Orange	42	4 oz	11
Peach	42	4 oz	11
Pear	38	4 oz	11
Pineapple	66	4 oz	10
Raisins	64	1/2 cup	44
Watermelon	72	4 oz	6
VEGETABLES			
Broccoli	15	1 cup	5
Cauliflower	15	1 cup	5
Carrots	47	1 cup	10
Corn	60	1/2 cup	18
Lettuce	15	1 cup	2
Peas	48	1/2 cup	10

(The New Glucose Revolution, by Jennie Brand-Miller is recommended for further values and understanding of the glycemic index.)

Meal Combinations

The glycemic index is extremely important to your dieting success. Some "nutritionists" don't place much value on this tool, and some don't even know it exists. Yet, it can be your greatest asset or your greatest enemy. Many individuals have enjoyed early dieting success with faultless nutrition and then unknowingly eaten a high-glycemic carb, only to be slammed with raging hunger and an insulin tailspin. I think we've all been there—four or five days into a "diet," we find ourselves at the bottom of a gallon of ice cream or lying on the couch with our pants unsnapped after an extended visit to a pizza buffet! Eating too many or the wrong kind of carbohydrates unleashes powerful hormonal reactions that even the strongest-willed often can't withstand.

Your own gastrointestinal system actually gives you a carbohydrate safety net, if you know how to use it properly. So far, I've given examples of low- and high-glycemic carb digestive pathways. The glycemic index is a continuum, however, and every food fits in somewhere. Obviously, staying as low as possible will offer the best results with the least "discomfort," but what if you really want a carb source that's not as low on the index as you wish it was? Protein and fat molecules are larger and denser than carbohydrates, and digesting them takes between one and three hours, sometimes longer. The valve (pyloric sphincter) between the stomach and small intestine will stay closed while digestion takes place, opening only one-to-three times per minute while the food is properly broken down. If you eat a carb source in combination with fat and protein sources, the carbohydrate gets caught up in the slowed digestive process. In short, a carb eaten alone will be digested and absorbed much faster than one eaten with fat and protein. Remember, slowed absorption of our carbs is a very good thing! We will revisit this concept after explanations of fat and protein.

(Figure 3:7) Sugar Saving Substitutions

Several sugar substitutes exist and may be used to replace sugar sources in cooking, baking, and general sweetening. Though tastes are individual, most artificial sweetener packets can replace two teaspoons of sugar. Non-calorie sweeteners include stevia, aspartame (Equal®), saccharin (Sweet 'N Low®), acesulfame K, and sucralose (Splenda®). My recommendation is stevia, an almost noncaloric sweetening agent derived from a cactus-like plant.

Sugar	Substitutes (packets)	Substitutes (bulk)
2 teaspoons	1 packet	1/2 teaspoon
1/4 cup	6 packets	3 teaspoons
1/3 cup	8 packets	4 teaspoons
1/2 cup	12 packets	6 teaspoons
3/4 cup	18 packets	9 teaspoons
1 cup	24 packets	12 teaspoons

Metabolic Transformation in Action

"I considered myself to be reasonably in shape and fit. After all, I still hit the gym most mornings. I had a personal trainer, lifted weights, did cardio, and basically followed a low fat diabetic diet. So, why was I still fat? Not awfully fat - just enough to make me feel self conscious in summer clothes. I didn't know how I could lose the ten to fifteen extra pounds. Spending more time exercising was out of the question and forget about eating less food - I was already hungry enough all the time! I was frustrated with the perpetual dieting and with the stubborn layer of fat that was covering my muscles. I was starting to believe that at 46 years old, maybe this was as good as it was going to get.

One of the trainers at the gym talked to me about his personal success with Dr. Joe and his *Metabolic Transformation Program.* Come on, I thought. I've read every diet book on the planet and know the calorie count and nutrition content of every food known to man. I figured I had the market cornered on what foods are healthy and what foods to stay away from - so what more could I possibly learn from this Dr. Joe? Nonetheless, I left with a brochure on Dr. Joe's program.

Apparently, this program generated weight loss and increased your metabolic rate while keeping blood sugar levels stable. This piqued my interest because I'm an insulin-dependent diabetic. Although I was following what was supposed to be a healthy diet, I couldn't get a handle on maintaining good blood sugar levels. Too high, too low, up and down - I felt like I was on a roller coaster. I wanted to get my diet under control.

I emailed Joe and he was very confident that he could help me achieve my goals. His enthusiasm gave me the hope I needed to get started. I couldn't wait to get my hands on his book and the literature.

It's tough to get rid of the "eat as little as possible" diet mentality and, at first, I was scared about having to eat every three or so hours because that seemed like I'd be eating a lot. I knew that in order to succeed, planning ahead and organization were key. I bit the bullet and made sure to pack and prepare meals in advance so that I would have the food I needed to eat for the next day. After a few days of eating this way and the resulting lack of constant hunger, I was hooked!

As Joe says, this was just the start. The real value to me was the day-to-day monitoring, seeing positive changes and learning during the

continued ⟶

Metabolic Transformation in Action

process. No one could lose the weight for me or force me to eat healthy, but I needed encouragement and I needed to be accountable to someone. Joe's vast knowledge, enthusiasm, and constant support were invaluable. Despite the numerous times I blew it (sometimes big time,) Joe never doubted I would ultimately succeed.

I've now almost reached my goals - my blood sugar has greatly improved and my diabetes is in good control. My weight is down and my muscles finally show! I truly feel great and look much better and leaner. I know that consistency will bring complete success and am extremely thankful to have had the opportunity to work with Joe."

Lyn, Import Manager

CHAPTER THREE KEY POINTS

➤ 1) Carbohydrates provide your body's primary source of energy. Limiting carbohydrates forces the body to use an alternative energy source: body fat.

➤ 2) High-glycemic carbs promote body fat creation, increased hunger, and decreased energy.

➤ 3) Low-glycemic carbs increase energy, decrease hunger, and help to avoid body fat storage as opposed to high-glycemic carbs .

➤ 4) Combining carbs with fat and protein further slows absorption of carbohydrates (refer to later chapter on Meal Planning.)

4

FAT

The Great Myth

"It is a well-known fact that to lose body fat, you have to eliminate dietary fat. Everyone knows that counting fat grams is the most important practice in losing fat. As a matter of fact, you can eat anything you want as long as you don't eat fat." Have you heard people say such things? Have you ever believed or do you presently believe them? These "opinions" have been accepted as facts for a long, long time. You will still find these ideas printed in nutrition textbooks. You already know I believe that carbohydrates are physiologically and practically the most important component in fat loss. Fat comes in a close second, but with it comes even more misconceptions and misinformation.

There is one main division of dietary fat: saturated and unsaturated. Saturated fats come most commonly from animal sources. Beef, pork, dairy products, eggs, and poultry contain saturated fats. Products made with these animal fats, such as butter, cream, and many others, are also saturated. Some choices have a great deal more or less than others. For example, fish, chicken, and turkey breast have dramatically less fat than does beef.

The problem with saturated fats lies primarily in their structure. They are much larger and more stable than unsaturated fats, and therefore much harder to break down. Since they don't break down easily, they circulate in the blood stream longer, create higher blood cholesterol levels, lead to atherosclerosis, and end up being stored in large portions as body fat. There really aren't many positive things to say about saturated fats.

Unsaturated fats are found mainly in plant sources such as olive oil, canola oil, flaxseed oil, grapeseed oil, borage oil, some nuts, and actually in some fish, like salmon. Molecularly, unsaturated fats are smaller, less stable, and easier to break down. Surprisingly, unsaturated fats actually have some unbelievably important health benefits and can help you lose body fat. Many unsaturated fats contain certain specific "essential fatty acids." Each essential fatty acid has unique properties and benefits to the human body. I will refer to unsaturated fats very generally in this text to simplify the content and stay true to our subject of body fat loss.

Good Fat?

Many people have heard the terms "good fat" and "bad fat." Looking just at the effects of fat on body composition, I can assure you that without unsaturated dietary fat, body fat loss will be slow at first, minimal at best, and ultimately counterproductive. Let me now explain these bold claims. Some essential fatty acids are the building blocks for certain hormones that control fat loss and storage, and the potential for muscle gain and loss. Reread that sentence. One more time, please…Yes, your body produces specific hormones that control how much body fat you can lose or gain and how much muscle you can gain or lose. Your body needs unsaturated fats (essential fatty acids) to create many of these hormones. As a matter of fact, many studies have confirmed this fact to be predictable and reproducible. In a matter of weeks, people who consume a no- or low-fat diet start producing less and less of the "good" hormones that promote body fat loss, as well as those that promote muscle gain. Conversely, people who consume 20 to 30 percent of their calories from unsaturated fat start producing more of these hormones, often above normal levels. With an increase in your hormonal base, you can actually burn more body fat than normal and build more muscle than normal. Studies have even shown incredibly positive blood chemistry changes, such as decreased cholesterol and increased athletic performance.

(Figure 4:1) Hormones

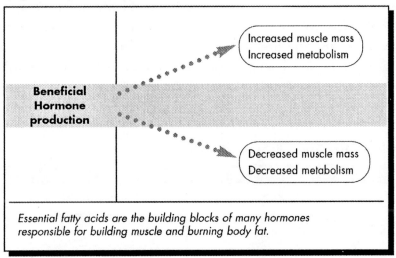

Increased muscle mass
Increased metabolism

Beneficial Hormone production

Decreased muscle mass
Decreased metabolism

Essential fatty acids are the building blocks of many hormones responsible for building muscle and burning body fat.

I have personally witnessed dramatic decreases in cholesterol and LDLs (bad fat in the bloodstream) by increasing total dietary fat. This can be achieved by eliminating saturated fats and increasing unsaturated fats while keeping carbs in check. You can't leave out carbohydrate control when discussing cholesterol.

Up to 80 percent of your body's cholesterol is produced in your liver as a result of sugar and runaway insulin. Remember that excess carbohydrates lead to a conversion to cholesterol and fat. By recommending higher intake of unsaturated fats while controlling carbohydrate levels, I have also witnessed hypercholesteremic clients (those whose livers produce a significantly larger amount of cholesterol) lower their cholesterol levels and manage them so well that, under the supervision of their physicians, they have been able to eliminate the use of cholesterol-reducing medications.

Another practical example of the power of correct nutrition is seen in elite athletes, whose body composition changes are easily measured and observed. I have personally consulted with and supervised the nutrition of hundreds of bodybuilders preparing for competition. They may need to lose between 15 and 40 pounds of body fat for the contest without losing muscle, and this can certainly be achieved. However, I have also tested the body composition of competitors that are not under my nutritional support, and I'm always amazed at how much muscle can be lost during dieting; quite a contrast to physiologically proper nutrition.

(Figure 4:2) Good Fats/Bad Fats

Unsaturated Fats:	Saturated Fats
*Easily used as energy	*Difficult to breakdown
*Decreases cholesterol	*Increases cholesterol
*Contains essential fatty acids	
*Necessary for many regenerative body processes	
*Essential fatty acids necessary to create certain hormones for optimal health, building muscle, and burning body fat	

Burgers and Oils

Consciously switching from saturated to unsaturated fats is a lot easier on paper than it is in real life. You can switch from a hamburger to a chicken breast, or from three whole eggs to six egg whites, but how are you going to get the good fats into your day? The most practical and healthy ways will be to add certain oils to your food. For example, if you have a bowl of oatmeal, add one half to a whole tablespoon of flax-seed oil after it's cooked. Do the same thing with brown rice, yogurt, protein shakes, or anything else that can withstand oil without destroying the taste of the food.

If you're making an egg white omelet, cook it with olive, canola, or grapeseed oil instead of a spray. If salad dressing is an area from which you get some of your fat intake, use an Italian dressing made with olive oil instead of a cream-based dressing with saturated fat. Almonds are a very healthy fat source that are very practical for a part of a snack. The longer you make better food choices, the more creative you'll become. Be patient and make the process fun, not overwhelming.

(Figure 4:3) Fatty Acid Composition (% of Total Fat) of selected oils:

	SF	OA	LA	GLA	ALA
Cooking Oils:					
Canola	7	54	30	0	7
Olive	16	76	8	0	0
Soy	15	26	50	0	9
Corn	17	24	59	0	0
Safflower	7	10	80	0	0
Medicinal Oils:					
Evening Primrose	10	9	72	9	0
Black Currant	7	9	47	17	13
Borage	14	16	35	22	0
Flax	9	19	14	0	58

SF = Saturated Fat
OA = Oleic Acid
LA = Linolenic Acid
GLA = Gamma-Linolenic Acid (omega - 6 oil)
ALA = Alpha-Linolenic Acid (omega - 3 oil)

(Taken from Understanding Fats and Oils, Dr. Michael T. Murray, N.D.)

Metabolic Transformation in Action

"What a blessing it's been to learn about life-changing nutrition from Joe Klemczewski! There aren't enough superlatives to describe him and his vast knowledge of nutrition and the human body. He genuinely cares about teaching people how to eat so our bodies can be as strong and healthy as God created them to be.

I had been active all my life in many different sports. I excelled in dance (mainly ballet,) swimming, aerobics, and karate. I never had to worry about what or how much I ate. It did not affect my weight.

In 1992 my food habits changed. I was eating out a lot and eating more of everything, especially sweets. I had moved to a new city and most of my athletic activities stopped. I jumped five sizes as my weight climbed. I had to do something. I altered what I was eating and started riding my bike and walking. Unfortunately, it wasn't working. My weight increased even more.

For a Christmas gift in 1999 my daughters gave me a gift certificate to Joe's gym. He suggested an appointment to talk about nutrition. Joe taught me that the body needs certain amounts of protein, carbohydrates, and good fat. I also learned I needed to eat six or seven times a day, maintaining these certain amounts that he suggested based on my body size and activity level. I wish anyone with a weight issue could learn what I did from Joe. The results will be good health and body leanness that can be enjoyed for the rest of life.

Because I followed Joe's plan, I immediately started losing weight. In just three months my weight was back where I wanted it. I was gaining muscle and had more energy. I was getting stronger and it felt great. With the weight under control and a commitment to continue exercising, I was able to maintain this accomplishment.

Looking back at those first days in the gym, I was so self-conscious of my legs rubbing together I would wear sweats to hide my legs and, yes, a tee shirt to hide the flab on my arms. Once I lost the weight I timidly wore workout shorts and a workout top in the gym. Someone said, "Tootie, where have you been hiding those muscles?!" Wow! What a mental boost! I felt

continued ———>

Metabolic Transformation in Action

like I had really accomplished something. That was the end of the cover-me-up clothes! It was the turning point in my training.

Joe made me feel like I was the only client he had. Taking a genuine interest in people, their accomplishments, and helping them achieve their goals, Joe is right there to take you to your maximum potential. After being exposed to some people in the gym and watching how hard they work to compete in bodybuilding and admiring their chiseled bodies, I set a never-before-imagined goal of doing the same.

This was something that I would love to have done in my twenties. Was it possible to do now at age 61? After talking to Joe, it was agreed. I would compete in the 2001 INBF Mid-America Muscle Classic Women's Grand Masters.

I was excited, a little nervous (actually petrified describes it best), but definitely determined. My training became more intense as did my determination. Besides lifting weights, we put a lot of time into selecting music, choreographing a routine, and practicing posing. I learned that behind every bodybuilder on stage there is a great, dedicated team. I had the very best. The encouragement of Joe, his staff, and even their families is awesome and contagious.

It has been amazing to learn from Joe that many of the nutrition ideas I thought to be factual were actually misconceptions that were working against me. I'm thankful Joe has been dedicated to putting his knowledge down on paper. His nutrition manual is the only one in my home. I put it to the test. It worked. Now I'm a 63-year-old woman with a body better than some 20 year olds. That's proof enough for me.

Share your ultimate goal with Joe, have the right attitude and determination, and he'll see that you achieve it. He encourages you beyond what you think your body is capable. I have complete faith and trust in Joe."

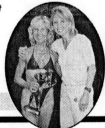

Tootie (with daughter, Dawndy), Realtor

A Little More Detail

A point that must be understood is how dynamic fat is in the body. If you gained 10 pounds last year, you're not retaining the exact same 10 pounds of body fat that was originally stored. Your body is constantly storing triglycerides in adipose (fat) cells and also releasing them as you need more energy between meals. In fact, adipose cells always store fat after meals and then release it when needed. Fat is actually used for up to 60 percent of the body's energy needs at rest A surprising point to most is how easily your body stores dietary fat as body fat. Dietary fat is the easiest nutrient for your body to store as body fat. As digested dietary fat is carried past adipose cells in the bloodstream through capillaries, adipose cells simply intake the fat to be stored.

If you're tracking this data carefully, you'll see why I stated that overall calorie intake is still always the first step. If you're taking in even a moderately low amount of fat, even unsaturated ("good") fats like flaxseed oil, a great deal of it can end up stored as fat. However, if your overall calorie intake is lower than your metabolic rate requires, you'll end up using that fat and "extra stored fat" between meals.

So, if so much of dietary fat ends up being stored as body fat, why not just eliminate it completely? The already discussed essential fatty acids found in certain unsaturated fats play a role in hormone production, cellular repair, immune function, and many other life processes. If one is deficient in these essential fatty acids, health consequences cumulatively add physical stress to the body. Another reason is the focus on keeping blood sugar moderated. Fat takes longer to digest and slows the digestion and assimilation of carbohydrates, so insulin spiking is less of a problem. This type of fat intake has merit, but only if the percentages are representative, once again, of an overall calorie intake that's low enough to cause a caloric deficit. The relationship between fat and carbohydrate intake is very important. If fat intake, for example, is 25 percent of the calorie intake instead of 15 percent, a little lower carbohydrate intake will be necessary to accommodate for the additional dietary fat. However, the lower carbohydrates may then make the practicality of food intake difficult, and energy levels may drop. Thus, a slightly lower fat intake, allowing for more carbohydrates, may be necessary. Some flexibility between carbohydrates and fat is allowed for in the suggested nutrient ranges table (Fig: 1:2), and you should feel comfortable trying different combinations as long as you stay within both ranges.

A discussion of fat intake and dietary theory wouldn't be complete without commenting on the ketogenic camp. What do we do with the experts that would have us eat unlimited amounts of fat and protein but eschew carbs with the promise of a shredded physique? Since excess carbs are easily converted to body fat and lead to lethargy, higher risk of diabetes and heart disease, and many other health perils, it's correct applied knowledge to control carbs and their quality. It's also imperative to make sure that carbs are low enough to not supply all the energy requirements of the body. A high-carb diet in which protein and fat intake is low will unlikely allow for much body fat loss because the body will have little reason to access a secondary energy source such as body fat. If you take the opposite extreme and eliminate almost all carbohydrates from the body, then stored fat will be released at a very rapid rate. Though seemingly used successfully by many bodybuilders, this type of dieting has its problems. First, adipose cells release fat to be used as energy in the form of glycerol and fatty acids. Body cells intake the glycerol and fatty acids to metabolize them into energy through the Kreb's cycle, but glucose fragments must be present. Let me repeat this: glucose fragments (carbs) must be present to burn body fat for energy through the very efficient Kreb's cycle within every cell; but it isn't the only way. If glucose isn't available, fatty acids can combine with each other to form ketone bodies that can also be used by most cells (with the exception of the brain's and nervous system's) for energy conversion. The rate of body fat usage for energy can be great using this method of diet, but the problems with this mechanism are many.

Ketogenic dieting may be effective only if fat intake isn't too excessive. Remember, adipose cells are just waiting to suck in new triglycerides to store after meals. The two greatest problems are that carbs are the most protein-sparing nutrient we eat. If carbs are too low for too long, you'll lose muscle no matter how much protein you eat, period! Also, the brain and nervous system can only use glucose, not ketone bodies, for energy. Low energy and less than optimal nervous system efficiency for muscle contractions leave workouts low-key, weak, and less effective. So, ketogenic dieting certainly allows you to burn more fat because of the immense carb deficit, but increasing fat intake too much can cause a great deal of fat storage. Two steps forward, two steps back. This, coupled with low energy workouts and muscle loss, isn't the best form of dieting. The few that have successfully employed this type of dieting, leave me wondering how much easier it would have been had they dieted "correctly."

So, what's the take-home message about fat? If you're in a maintaining, isocaloric stage of non-dieting, you can successfully eat 30 percent or more of your calories from fat sources without a problem—though I would chose approximately 20 percent so more protein and/or carbs can be consumed. The key is in the word "isocaloric," or eating the same amount of total calories that your body uses for energy so that whatever ratios you chose, you won't store new body fat. If you're dieting to a very low level, you can save yourself from taking too many steps backward by cutting fat intake to 10-15 percent of total calories. This simply means less fat will be available for storage after meals and the amount of stored fat used between meals for energy will be coming from a faster shrinking supply. Going lower, however, will trigger the metabolic ill effects of too low a fat intake. Carbohydrate control and planning is just as important as dietary fat, but in reality the two go hand-in-hand. Many people that obsess about carbs alone end up snacking on nuts, peanut butter, and other high-fat, low-carb foods, only to increase direct fat storage from the increased fat intake. When taking in a limited amount of fat, be sure to make the most of what you get and supplement with essential fatty acid containing unsaturated fats. Don't lose sight of the big picture, however: Dietary fat intake is a critical part of your success, but it has to be just one piece of a perfect comprehensive plan to work!

One last word about fats: Have a steak once in awhile. A small percentage of saturated fat isn't going to throw you into cardiac arrest, and if your cholesterol is actually too low, you can suffer from low energy, low hormonal levels, and even depression.

Fat Reducing Tips

1) Use non-stick cooking spray to reduce fat or use unsaturated oils to increase "good" fat when cooking.

2) Boil, roast, bake, or steam food in place of frying.

3) Use egg whites in place of whole eggs when baking. 2 egg whites equal one whole egg.

4) Use skim milk in place of whole or 2% milk.

5) Choose low or no-fat yogurts, mayo, and salad dressings.

6) Use spices and fat-free condiments such as salsa to spice up food.

7) Use applesauce in place of butter and/or oil in baked goods.

8) Make sure canned tuna, chicken, and other meats are packed in water, not oil.

9) Chose the leanest cuts of meat.

10) Trim fat from meat.

CHAPTER FOUR KEY POINTS

1) Saturated fats are found primarily in animal sources.

2) Saturated fats lead to heart disease and body fat.

3) Unsaturated fats contain essential fatty acids that are necessary for many body processes.

4) Unsaturated fats in the right amounts are necessary to lose the maximal amount of body fat and to build muscle.

5

PROTEIN

So Many Choices!

Just as most saturated fats come from animal sources, so does protein. Uh oh, now we have a problem. We need protein, but we don't want saturated fat. Luckily, God made some pretty lean animals. Fish, chicken and turkey breast, ostrich, egg whites, and even soy-based meat substitutes offer an alternative to foods high in saturated fats like beef, pork, dairy products, and whole eggs. These healthier foods are now commonly found on the menus of most restaurants, meaning they're easy to obtain on the go.

Another convenient protein choice comes in the form of protein powders, shakes, and bars. The reason professional athletes endorse supplement companies (besides getting paid) is that they actually use their products. It can be a lot easier to get supplemental protein in the form of a great tasting shake or bar, especially in on-the-run situations. I couldn't eat properly and still see a high volume of patients and clients without an occasional bar or shake to supplement my whole-food meals. Getting some of your protein from sources like shakes and bars will also help you avoid the "I'll-puke-if-I-eat-another-chicken-breast" syndrome.

Why Protein?

Most bodybuilders would correctly tell you that you need protein to build muscle. They would probably also tell you, however, that you need two-to-three times what you really require. If you asked a vegetarian about protein, you might learn how to make a dozen eggs last for a year. Your body has the ability to survive either extreme, but you will pay the price for each. You can survive without much protein at all, but you will strip the muscle right off your bones and impair your ability to build the healthiest cells. Too much protein, as advocated by some muscle magazines (owned by protein supplement companies), and you may spend a lifetime in a state of acidosis (creating a host of degenerative diseases) or, according to registered dieticians, you could end up on the kidney transplant waiting list. So, how much is best?

(Figure 5:1) Protein Utilization

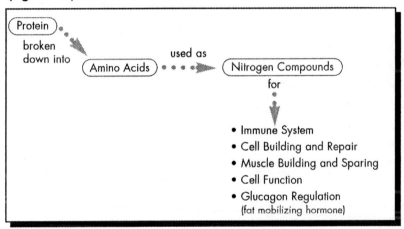

The amounts of protein I advocate are designed to abundantly meet the body's requirements without the risk of undesirable effects. Protein is very important in creating new cells, such as red blood cells, skin cells, liver cells, etc., as well as in the maintenance and metabolic activities of every system in your body. If protein intake is too low, your entire body suffers eventually, even your immune system. At first, you can withstand protein depletion very efficiently because you have so much stored. Protein is broken down into amino acids, which are used in just about every chemical reaction that takes place within your body. Amino acids are made up of nitrogen compounds that circulate in your bloodstream and are stored in a few places, mostly as skeletal muscle, and some in the liver. So yes, you can live a long time without protein, and even longer with insufficient amounts of protein; your body will simply break down your muscle tissue to provide what it needs. It's a great survival mechanism, but as far as I'm concerned, I don't want to knowingly lose any muscle, and neither should you.

I estimate protein requirements for active people. If you aren't performing rigorous exercise at least three-to-four times per week, chose the lower end of suggested protein ranges (Chapter One). If you perform extremely high amounts of training per week, you may actually need to go slightly above my suggestions.

Variety is the Spice of Life

Every protein has a specific amino acid profile. This means each protein source may be higher or lower in certain amino acids than other protein sources. There are many rating scales that attempt to build a hierarchy among protein sources by assigning values and deeming them "high-" or "low-"quality protein sources. There is merit to these types of ratings. However, even the highest-rated protein source is low in certain amino acids, and lower-rated proteins have higher levels of specific amino acids than the top proteins.

You may have also heard that you have to combine certain proteins to "complete the amino acid chain." You're covered on this one on two different fronts. First, digestion, absorption, and circulation keeps the amino acids that you consume available for hours, and they can be augmented with other amino acids in previous or later meals. The liver also stores a small reserve of amino acids that it uses when necessary.

The bottom line, therefore, is simply to enjoy a variety of protein sources throughout your day. Keep in mind: Saturated fats should be kept to a minimum so that your diet leaves room for high-quality unsaturated fats and essential fatty acids.

Metabolic Transformation in Action

"I have been eating disordered, in one way or another, my entire life. My earliest memories all involve food. I remember downing the entire contents of the sugar bowl that sat on our kitchen table. I must have been 3 or 4 years old.

I was a chubby kid and put on my first diet by my pediatrician in second grade. I did so well the first week that my mom took me out for ice cream as a reward! The diet soon fell by the wayside, as did the countless diets that followed.

My weight yo-yoed up and down all through junior high. I would go on starvation diets only to follow them with periods of binging. In high school I found what I thought was the cure to my weight problems. AMPHET-AMINES! (You have to remember that this was the seventies and everyone did drugs). It was now easier to starve myself. I would just replace my drug of choice (food) with any other substance I could get my hands on. I would lose twenty pounds in a week only to put it back on when I came crashing down. I continued off and on this drug enhanced weight loss method for about twelve years. At the end of that time, I tipped the scales at 190.

Then Oprah found the liquid diet and so did I. I lost fifty pounds in just a few months. It also led me to my next weight loss method, vomiting. The liquid diet shrank my stomach (albeit temporarily) and I couldn't handle the binges. I was very proud of myself and thought that this was great. I would now be able to eat whatever I wanted and still not get fat. How cool was that?

I managed to keep my weight fairly stable for a few years. When I finally gave up purging, my weight started to balloon upwards again. Within a few years I weighed 242.

Then came the next great weight loss method. Phen-fen! It was amazing! For the first time in my life, I actually felt like the compulsion was gone. I lost ninety pounds. This only lasted a short time. No one told me that you get used to the drugs. I was still hanging on and then the unimaginable; the FDA banned the drug!!

I totally gave up and gave in to my addiction and within a year I had once again gained back all the weight plus some. Within 3 years I was at my all time high, 265 pounds.

continued ⟶

Metabolic Transformation in Action

I functioned (or pretended to function) at this weight for about two years. It was really starting to take a toll. I ached everywhere. I was really worried that I was going to die and hoped that it would happen soon. Looking for the magic cure once again, I considered stomach surgery, even knowing that two out of every hundred die from the procedure. Luckily, I'm cheap and my insurance wouldn't pay for it.

I knew that it was now or never. I was either going to lose the weight or die. I went on the liquid diet yet again and lost fifty pounds. That was enough motivation to join a gym. I started weight training and doing cardio. I was really motivated and the weight continued to come off. In nine months I had lost 115 pounds and weighed 150 pounds. Now what was I going to do? How the heck was I going to continue to lose/maintain and eat at the same time? Impossible!!!!

I managed to lose a few more pounds and hit a wall. I would stay on my eating plan that I devised for myself for a few days and then give in to the overwhelming urge to binge. I knew that if I didn't do something, I would gain all the hard lost weight back. That's when I met Dr. Joe.

I went to a seminar where Dr. Joe was speaking about nutrition for competitive bodybuilders. He finally made sense out of science. I have read every diet book known to mankind but none was as clear cut and made as much sense as what I was hearing from this man, my new hero. I asked Dr. Joe to work with me so that I could get to and maintain my goal weight. He gave me my nutrient numbers and helped me do the work. Joe monitored my diet via e-mail.

Within two months I had dropped that last twelve pounds and had attained my goal of losing half my body weight. Believe it or not (I still have trouble wrapping my brain around this one), I decided that I had gotten a little too thin and intentionally put a few pounds back on. I've never had to gain weight in my life!!

Because of my physical and emotional addiction to food, I had never before attained a weight loss goal. I have always done something to sabotage myself. I now know that there is no magic pill, no cure. Although it's science, it's not rocket science. Joe has laid it all out in a manner that any

continued ———▶

Metabolic Transformation in Action

> one can follow. To this day, I still have my ups and downs but with Dr. Joe's help, I intend to maintain my svelte new figure and finally wrestle my evil fat twin to her blubbery demise."
>
> Liz, Accounting Consultant

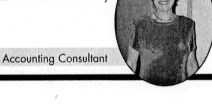

Back to Hormones

Just as carbohydrates can affect your body in a positive or negative way through the modulation of the hormone insulin, protein creates a similar affect through the hormone glucagon. Insulin is a storage hormone; it shuttles glucose into cells and corrals excess amounts of it to the liver to be converted into body fat. To oversimplify, insulin is released when you eat carbs; glucagon is released when you eat protein. Just as insulin is a storage hormone, glucagon is a retrieval, or mobilizing, hormone. It actually promotes glucose to be used as energy, and when glucose isn't present in large enough quantities (because you've been so good at limiting your carbs and sticking to your daily totals!) it helps mobilize body fat to be burned as energy. Hence the importance of breaking your daily macronutrient totals up so that you can have protein in most meals. Think of insulin and glucagon as representing two opposite metabolic stimuli. Insulin is present, active, and dominant if carbohydrate intake is too high, and your body is thus in a storage mode. Glucagon is more dominant when carbohydrate intake is lower and protein intake is higher, promoting fat mobilization. Glucagon is one of several hormones that can "unlock" body fat cells, but is the most powerful that is nutrition-dependent. Others are more exercise-dependent.

Protein also has the greatest "thermic potential" among macronutrients. This means that when you eat protein, your metabolism raises because its digestion requires more energy. Protein is very important for health and body composition, but in most cases it is deficient in American diets. This, along with hormonal considerations such as glucagon, is the reason many new studies are showing that diets higher in protein and lower in carbs can cause twice as much body fat loss—even with the same amount of calories!

CHAPTER FIVE KEY POINTS

1) Protein is found in animal meats and sometimes in small amounts in certain beans and plants.

2) Supplemental protein can be found in many types of protein shakes and bars.

3) Protein is necessary for many vital processes in the body as well as muscle growth.

4) Protein sources have different amino acid profiles, making it advantageous to vary your protein choices.

5) Eating protein raises your metabolism and through the actions of the hormone glucagon assists you in losing body fat faster.

6

MEAL RATIOS

Better Living through Chemistry

Few authors or "experts" have ever validated their "diets" with actual research. The reason we have been tossed to and fro, from one diet to another, is that they promise great results, but unfortunately their diets are physiologically unverified. For the average person, nutrition is often a black hole of mystery and marketing. Only recently have scientists started conducting thorough research on food's affect on health and body composition. Believe it or not, there are still highly trained experts, even medical doctors, that think what you eat doesn't matter. One pioneer in food research, Dr. Barry Sears, Ph.D., would disagree. The mantra throughout his *Zone Diet* series is that food is the greatest "drug" affecting our bodies.

Before many "diet" books were ever published, my bodybuilding career was well underway, and I was experimenting with different forms of dieting. My education and self-studying led me to metabolic physiology and away from the fad diets in magazines. While my peers were still blindly following high-carb, low-fat diets and no-carb, high fat diets, I was incorporating what I deduced was necessary for optimal body function via medical and nutritional textbooks. As my nutritional understanding evolved, my personal results were amazing, and my contest dieting and preparation reached new levels. While I was stumbling upon a greater understanding of nutrition from a physiological perspective, some biochemistry-oriented researchers were perfecting it clinically. More information emerged refuting the carbohydrate dominant, low-protein, low-fat diets thought to be best for dieting and performance. I was ecstatic, since it paralleled my practical understanding and affirmed my theories with hard, irrefutable science. Combining this science with the individuality of body types and the variables of individuals' lifestyles has led to amazing results for my clients.

Measuring Cups and Calculators

Reviewing much of what we've discussed already will help to pull this section together. Eating the right amount of food per day and breaking that food into small meals are the first steps in creating your eating structure. We have also established the importance of every macronutrient and the best choices of each. The point was also made that each macronutrient needs to be consumed in each meal. In other words, carbs, fat, and protein should be eaten together in small, evenly spaced meals throughout the day, in amounts that will keep us in our daily intake ranges. The big questions, then, are: Do I have to have the same amount of protein, carbs, and fat in each meal? And do I have to have the same ratios of nutrients in each meal?

Let me preface the following explanation with the answer "yes and no." To allow some flexibility, I suggest a small range in each macronutrient rather than a rigid amount of food per meal or per day. I'll explain my rationale, but first let me offer that once you are locked into a "normal" eating pattern within your daily totals, you will achieve the best results if your meals represent an even distribution of macronutrients throughout the day. Sixty grams of carbs in one meal and 10 in the next just isn't going to cut it. You want a good ratio of nutrients in each meal.

Metabolic Transformation in Action

"All of my adult life I have been overweight despite being very active. I was not able to slim down. I was 35 years old, 5'5" and weighed 173 pounds. I ran a marathon at that weight! I couldn't understand how I could run, run, run and not lose a single pound! I was very concerned about my weight. I had just accepted a new job that would require me to travel for several days or weeks at a time; what was I going to do now? I thought for sure that I would be over 200 pounds by Christmas! I had a sense of urgency to do something but was not sure where to start. All the dieting I had done in the past was not working for me now. I was depressed and desperate.

It began. My journey that is. A newspaper ad, a money back guarantee to lose weight, and a phone call to Dr. Joe. I made an appointment and Dr. Joe went systematically over all of the steps of the program I was to start. The pounds started melting away. My husband was thrilled with the new me and so was I.

Suddenly one day I was startled to notice that my neck felt weird and tight. The pain was crippling a times; it interrupted my concentration, my sleep, my weight training, my running, and most of all my eating. After four months of physical therapy, a wagonload of prescription drugs, and several tests, I was facing a major surgery. My first thought was, "Why me?" I had lost 35 pounds!

Four months after my surgery I returned to weightlifting and running. I avoided the scales since my surgery and was getting curious as to how much weight I had gained back. Much to my surprise, I weighed the same as I did before the surgery! How was this possible?! At times during my recovery, it seemed I was eating everything in sight, however, when I realized that wasn't going to help anything, I returned to what Joe had taught me.

Currently, I have lost a total of 60 pounds. Without the nutritional guidance of Dr. Joe, my success now and in the future would not be possible. Thanks, Joe, for your guidance and encouragement!"

Jennifer, Loan Analyst

There are, however, times when some flexibility is not only helpful, but simply the right thing to do. For example, if you've just performed an intense workout, your next meal may include a little higher percentage of carbohydrates to refill the stored glycogen (sugar) used in the muscle tissue. If you're going to bed soon, and you're hungry, it would be better to have a higher percentage of protein and less carbs. This will actually stimulate more growth hormone to be released at night and suppress insulin, which inhibits growth hormone. You will also find that you're hungrier during some points of the day than you are at others. You may need a small meal only two hours after eating during the morning, but you can go three hours after lunch. Some meals will be larger, and some smaller. The point is, flexibility is often helpful due to schedules, is often physiologically necessary, and can help with your own compliance to succeed with this new eating pattern. There is a balance, however, between what is right and perfect nutritionally, and the level you can achieve in your daily life. I have provided the ranges to give you this flexibility day-to-day and meal-to-meal, but you still have to be responsible for implementing this plan consistently.

CHAPTER SIX KEY POINTS

1) Keep nutrient totals as evenly spaced throughout meals as possible.

2) Allow yourself flexibility when necessary regarding meal ratios but stay within your nutrient totals for the day.

3) Keep meal spacing as even as possible with two to four hours between meals and snacks.

4) Learn your body's natural hunger patterns and adjust meal spacing accordingly, allowing for some flexibility.

7

RECIPES AND FOOD PREPARATION

Just Tell Me What to Eat!

Most new clients sit across from me in full trust, expecting body fat loss and positive health changes similar to what they have seen in the person that referred them to me. Occasionally, however, someone tries to help me by offering feedback on my information or methods of delivery. I have learned a great deal and invite all the criticism and feedback that clients are willing to give, but there is one common request I always refuse. A mild version of this request is a client that asks for recipes and meal plans, and that hints at wanting the inclusion of an entire daily menu. The more severe version comes from clients that beg for a written menu to follow, or simply "won't be able to succeed." "I promise, just tell me what to eat and I'll eat it! I don't care if I eat the same thing every meal, every day!"

For this client, I predict failure. This is a client that has tried everything else and has failed more as a result of lacking initiative and discipline than due to a faulty nutrition plan. Though it seems easier, you don't want to follow a meal-by-meal plan written by me or anyone else. Nobody knows what foods you like, what your schedule is like, or what challenges may be unique to you. You have to learn to interact with food, any food, and put it into your daily plan successfully. I have provided a small amount of meal samples for you to view as examples; however, my goal is for you to create your own food intake based on the nutritional values proposed in chapter one.

When a client comes to me through a class, a consultation, or my online program, I purposely make the first step one of personal menu planning. My client goes home and figures out what he or she is going to eat the next day, making the best food choices, keeping nutrient totals and meal spacing as even as possible, and creating four-to-six meals that fall into the suggested nutrient ranges. Yes, it takes a food-count book, a calculator, an eraser, and a lot of patience. Once you've taken this step, however, you are well on your way to success, because you have a framework from which to build a pattern. You will quickly learn to substitute a variety of food and meal choices and stay within your plan. Without this planning, you will likely not be able to continue with your plan. The responsibility I ask my clients to assume is the driving force that makes the science of nutrition elements work. My clients learn to adapt, be creative, and begin an ongoing process of cumulative learning. They become their own best nutritionists. They succeed.

Yet, many people that join a "weight loss center" end up gaining back all the lost weight within one year. These chain weight loss centers pride themselves on making it easy for their customers by giving them diet plans, meal cards, follow-along daily menus, and even prepackaged food. On this issue, I gladly walk 180 degrees in the opposite direction. Studies have determined that the majority of the people that engage in these programs weigh more one year later than the day they walked in the door. The initial ease offered by a menu is quickly complicated by the fact that you have a different schedule, different tastes, different goals, and different metabolic needs than everyone else. Secondly, you simply learn nothing about nutrition and how to make permanent changes unless you go through a progressive learning process.

What's That?

There are already plenty of good recipe books out there. I simply want to provide examples that show how you can create a day of good meals within your proposed food amount for the day. It begins with your realization that eating the right foods in the right amounts is your focus. You don't have to make a meal for your family and a separate meal for yourself. Simply take the right foods in the right amounts. This leads to why I devalue recipes slightly. You don't have to have elaborate recipes and exotic ingredients, or even "special" foods, to diet and eat correctly. Right foods, right amounts. I can throw a can of tuna in a bowl with a cup of brown rice, stir in a half a tablespoon of flax-seed oil, pour on some salsa, and I'm ready to eat. Breakfast? No problem! Mix a scoop of strawberry protein powder into my already cooked 1/2-cup of oatmeal and add some almonds or oil, and I'm off to the office. Creativity! You may get some funny looks once in awhile, but you'll have the last laugh.

Breakfast without Sugar

Most breakfast selections are a disastrous way to start your day. Sugar and refined (high-glycemic) flour is used to create very tasty cereals, as long as you don't mind a little extra body fat, low energy, and hunger. You're not a cereal person? How about a doughnut or a "healthier" refined-flour bagel with 50 grams of carbs? Breakfast bars, pastries—yep, same story.

Breakfast is actually a difficult meal for most people due to time constraints and/or a lack of food ideas. Unless you want my tuna and salsa concoction for breakfast, I suggest a little planning. Protein is difficult unless you have time to cook egg white combinations or utilize a protein substitute. Scrambled egg whites (with one whole egg, if you like, and the extra fat fits in your meal plan) cooked in olive or canola oil, joined by oat or rye toast, make a great breakfast. You can even get fancy with different omelets.

Oatmeal (watch for added sugar in flavored brands) is an excellent choice and can be fortified with fat and protein, as noted earlier. Meal replacement shakes can also be very helpful. These are protein powders packaged in individual servings (or simply use a protein powder), and they make great shakes in a blender where you can add your choice of high-quality oil and low-glycemic fruit, if your daily totals warrant. You can't get much quicker than that.

Food Source	Protein	Carbs	Fat
3 egg whites	12	0	0
1 piece whole grain toast	2	13	1
1 tsp. Canola oil	0	0	4
(to cook eggs)			
Total	14	13	5
(Great light breakfast that is very balanced and from filling whole foods.)			
6 egg whites/ 1 yolk	27	0	6
2 pieces whole grain toast	4	26	2
1 tsp. Canola oil	0	0	4
Totals	31	26	12
(Similar breakfast but larger.)			
1/2 cup (dry) oats	5	27	3
1 scoop protein powder	30	5	1
1/2 tbsp. Flaxseed oil	0	0	6
Totals	35	32	10
Mix powder and oil into oats after oats are cooked.			
(Protein powder is optional but does significantly fortify this already great breakfast.)			
1/2 cup low-fat cottage cheese	13	4	5
4 egg whites	16	0	0
1 tsp. Canola oil (to cook)	0	0	4
Chopped omelet veggies	0	3	0
Totals	29	7	9
Mix cottage cheese and egg whites in bowl, then make omelet.			
(High protein, low carb breakfast that is versatile and tastes great.			
Add carb sources such as toast if desired.)			

Food Source	Protein	Carbs	Fat
1/2 cup low-fat, plain yogurt	8	10	2
1 scoop protein powder	30	5	1
1/8 cup almonds	3	3	7
1/4 cup (dry) oats	3	13	1
Totals	44	31	11

Mix everything together into yogurt. May substitute high-fiber cereal for oats.
May add fruit for more carbs if needed.
Cut in half if necessary for your meal plan.
(This quick option tastes like dessert for breakfast!)

Food Source	Protein	Carbs	Fat
Meal replacement shake	40	20	1
1/2 tbsp. Flaxseed oil	0	0	5
8 oz. Skim milk	8	4	2
Totals	48	24	8

May substitute 1 tbsp. Peanut butter for flaxseed oil. May use water instead of milk.
Blend in mixer with ice. May use scoop of protein powder instead of meal
replacement packet to decrease protein and carbs.
(This is a quick but significant jump-start for the day.)

Food Source	Protein	Carbs	Fat
1 cup high-fiber cereal	3	35	1
1 cup skim milk	8	4	2
1/2 scoop protein powder	15	2	1
Totals	26	41	4

Mix vanilla protein powder well in milk, pour on cereal.
(Can't get much faster than this, but measure well; the carbs in cereal add up fast!)

Food Source	Protein	Carbs	Fat
3 egg whites	12	0	0
3 pieces low-fat turkey bacon	9	0	3
1 tsp. Canola oil (to cook)	0	0	4
2 pieces whole grain toast	4	26	2
Totals	25	26	9

May use whole grain pancakes instead of toast. May drop 1 piece of toast to
decrease carbs. May make into sandwich.
(If you have time, this is a classic!)

Lunch and Supper the Easy Way

Lunch and supper, or even whole food snacks, can easily be pieced together by combining compatible protein, carbohydrate, and fat choices. Choose your protein source and then add complimentary carbs and fat. If it's a chicken breast, decide whether you want pasta, brown rice, a sweet potato—it's your choice. Add a small healthy fat source—if necessary—to reach your suggested nutrient amounts for your meal plan and eat. A deli (chicken or turkey breast) sandwich can be made with low-glycemic bread and condiments. Health food stores even have mayonnaise made with canola oil instead of saturated fat! A chicken breast salad with a little Italian dressing is a great choice. The salad vegetables give you great carbs and the dressing gives you olive oil. Your creativity and planning are the only factors that can inhibit you from enjoying great tasting food and easy-to-prepare meals.

Food Source	Protein	Carbs	Fat
5 oz. Chicken breast	35	0	5
1/2 cup rice	2	22	0
Salad or can of green beans	0	10	0
2 tbsp. low/no-fat dressing	0	2	2
Totals	37	34	7

(This is a "full-size" lunch or supper that is complete in all categories.)

Food Source	Protein	Carbs	Fat
4 oz. Deli turkey breast	28	0	4
2 pieces whole grain bread	4	26	2
Lettuce/tomato	0	0	0
Mustard	0	0	0
Totals	32	26	6

May use 1 piece of bread to decrease carbs and add a small salad to increase fiber.
(A "plain 'ole sandwich" can be a great meal.)

Food Source	Protein	Carbs	Fat
4 oz. Tuna	30	0	0
1 tbsp. Light Miracle Whip	0	2	3
Small salad (varies)	0	10	0
5 small whole wheat crackers	0	10	2
Totals	30	22	5

(Quick and easy tuna salad.)

Food Source	Protein	Carbs	Fat
3 oz. Chicken breast strips	21	0	3
1 tortilla wrap (varies)	0	5	1
Lettuce, veggie condiments	0	5	0
3-4 tbsp salsa (varies)	0	5	0
Totals	21	15	4

(Creative and delicious!)

Food Source	Protein	Carbs	Fat
Chicken breast sandwich/sub	30	35	5

Estimate well or look up in a food count book.
Ask for no mayo, no cheese.
(Everyone's on the go sometimes!)

Food Source	Protein	Carbs	Fat
Meal replacement shake	40	20	1
Mixed in water			
(Not the preferable whole food lunch, but quick in a pinch.)			
Protein Bar (varies)	30	30	7
(Best used as a snack so you can get fiber and whole food meals, but in an emergency...)			
Small salad (varies)	0	10	0
1/2 cup low-fat cottage cheese	13	4	5
Pop-top can of chicken	13	0	1
Totals	26	14	6
(Just a quick, small lunch option.)			
4 oz. Baked fish	24	0	1
1 cup steamed broccoli	0	8	0
4 oz. Baked potato	1	30	0
1 tsp. Butter	0	0	5
Totals	25	38	6
(A great pattern for dinner.)			
1/2 oz. Almonds	3	3	6
3 oz. Chicken	21	0	3
1 TBSP Miracle Whip Light	0	2	3
Dash of Curry (spice)	0	0	0
2 Pieces Whole Wheat Bread	6	24	0
Totals	30	29	12
(Any recipe can be used as long as the amounts of foods used are measured and tracked. Be creative!!)			

Snacks

Snacks are vital to your plan. They keep your blood chemistry stable (as long as your food choices are appropriate), lessen hunger, help to keep you from overeating at meals, and keep your metabolism high. Convenience, however, can compromise quality if you're not careful. To keep food quality high, snacks may be an area where you need to be more flexible with the spacing of your nutrients. For example, an apple and 1/8 cup of almonds would make a great snack of low-glycemic carbs and quality fat, but the protein is low. Making sure your protein was adequate at your previous and your next meals would therefore be imperative. There are also a few high-quality snack bars that have a balanced amount of protein, carbs, and fat. I depend on these a great deal. They are especially good when you crave chocolate or dessert flavors, since there are many great flavors out there.

After-dinner snacks can consist of a small amount of crackers—one serving per package, popcorn, protein shake, etc. Try to keep under 150-200 calories per late-night snack. Weight loss will be accelerated if after-dinner snacking is eliminated or minimized.

Food Source	Protein	Carbs	Fat
Meal replacement shake Mixed in water	40	20	1
Protein Bar (varies)	30	30	7
1 Scoop Protein Powder	30	5	0
1/2 C Skim Milk	4	5	0
1/2 C Pineapple	0	15	0
1 C Strawberries	1	11	0
1 tsp. Flax Seed Oil	0	0	4
Totals	35	36	5
(Add ice, blend, freeze, and thaw out about one hour before eating. Tastes like frozen yogurt. Or, just blend and drink!)			
1/2 C Skim Milk	4	5	0
1/2 Scoop Protein Powder	15	2	0
1 TBSP Peanut Butter	5	4	8
Totals	24	11	8
(You can make an infinite variety of protein shakes!)			
"Energy/snack" bar	16	24	8
Apple	1	30	0
(Yep, just an apple can be fine. Watch out though, as a stand-alone carb source you may get hungry soon after.)			
Yogurt (per label)	10	20	3

Surviving Restaurants

1) Specify how you want food prepared to avoid added butter, etc.

2) Order baked, grilled, or broiled entrees.

3) Ask for salad dressings on the side (fat-free if possible.)

4) Share a meal.

5) Ask for grilled or steamed veggies instead of potato or rice if reducing carbohydrates.

6) Use red sauces instead of cream sauces.

7) Ask for cheese, croutons, bacon, egg yolks, and nuts to be left off salad.

8) Dip fork in dressing instead of pouring dressing on salad.

9) Ask for complimentary bread or chips to not be brought to the table.

10) Use a food count book to plan and estimate food intake.

CHAPTER SEVEN KEY POINTS

1) The right foods in the right amounts should be your focus.

2) You can construct fancy recipes, but this is unnecessary. Be creative and plan ahead using foods you like.

3) Did I mention, "Be creative"?

8

PUTTING IT ALL TOGETHER

Does it Really Work?

You can take the most important step to ensure your success right now. When a client leaves my office for the first time, I can predict his or her success with indescribable accuracy. I'm not a prophet; I'm a scientist. I observe patterns and trends as people interact with science and life. I see people succeed and I see people fail. The best and most accurate information means nothing if you don't or can't apply it. My clients that take the initiative here never fail. This first step is critical: It is simply to start now. Use the Six Week Program Guide (or your own notebook) and start recording your food intake <u>now</u>. Waiting until tomorrow will lead you to next week, next week will lead you to failure, and you may just throw away your last chance to gain total control over food, your health, and your physique. Start today. Record everything you eat for a day or two as you make small changes that you easily recall from this book. Start fine-tuning your nutrition by making better-quality food choices, improving your meal spacing, concentrating on meal ratios, and reaching your target macronutrient totals. Adjust your nutrient totals as described, if necessary, so that you are losing one-to-two pounds per week. Before you know it, you'll be feeling better than you thought possible, losing weight, and you'll be well on your way to becoming your own nutritionist.

Guaranteed?

It's hard for me not to guarantee absolute success to everyone, because I know that absolute success is possible for everyone. The greatest deterrent to your success once you get started is reaching too high of a comfort level too soon. I occasionally have a client that starts with the incredible motivation that comes with the new understanding of nutrition. This client starts losing two-to-three pounds a week, refers friends to our facility, and is ecstatic with the results. This client meticulously documents food and nutrient totals and consistently progresses. Then one day, progress slows; sometimes the client starts regaining weight. All of a sudden, either "it's just not working anymore" or they suddenly "have a slow metabolism." I ask to see the client's nutrition journal, and the reply is often, "Well, I quit writing things down last month." Translation: "I've lost my motivation. I'm cheating. In short, I'm no longer doing what needs to be done."

As soon as this client gets back on track—guess what? Their results pick right up where they left off. The point of this drawn-out example is that you must be consistent to reach your goal. It is so easy to slip upwards into "maintenance" eating. You're still eating perhaps the right percentages of macronutrients, but add just a little too much food and the intake volume may take you out of the losing range and into the maintenance range. My advice would be to stick with your weight-loss level of food intake for as long as you can and then take a planned break where you increase your volume to a maintenance level to "catch your breath," regroup, and then go right back to progressing. I can't emphasize enough that your initial progress and understanding needs to be underlined by consistency.

Prepare to Win!

Once you've gotten off to a great start, prepare for a long journey of experimentation, changes, new understanding, and better integration of proper nutrition into your daily life. I know it's a cliché, but these changes should be lifestyle changes. A shift in your thought processes regarding food has to occur. It is incredibly rewarding for me to see a client lose the 34th and 35th pounds, or to have a client reach the goal of losing 15 pounds in eight weeks. However, I'm ecstatic when I see that client enjoying a higher quality of life a year later—without having gained any weight back. This long-term success has very little to do with me. I take great joy in knowing that clients took the right information and worked hard and consistently to win what were perhaps great wars in their lives. I can educate and motivate, I can encourage and help with adjustments, but ultimately it's you that will or will not succeed. We may all fall down once in awhile, but not all of us get back up. As the initial motivation wears off and the ice cream is no longer as easy to pass on, you have to remember who you're doing this for. I know you can do it!

CHAPTER EIGHT KEY POINTS

• • • ▶ 1) Start right now!

• • • ▶ 2) Document meticulously.

• • • ▶ 3) Consistency, consistency, consistency.

• • • ▶ 4) It doesn't matter how many times you fall down, only how many times you get back up!

• • • ▶ 5) You're in this for life - be patient and enjoy the trip!

• • • ▶ 6) Prepare your mind for battle; prepare to win!!

9

SIX WEEKS TO METABOLIC TRANSFORMATION

Let's Get Started!!

Most of my clients have attended a lecture or a one-on-one consultation with me and then received a copy of the original manuscript of this book. I have observed countless reactions from them, and this has helped me refine my approach to help them and you to be more successful. I see a lot of "eureka" moments as clients start to understand past errors and connect all the dots of sound nutrition. Rarely does a client leave without ecstatically thinking they've found the missing link and then beginning their new program with great confidence. Rarely, however, do they start without getting overwhelmed by the sheer volume of new information. This six-week start is an incredible tool that will cement all the physiology you find on these pages into your eating habits—one step at a time! Following this six-week program has become as close to a 100 percent guarantee for your success as anything I have ever seen.

Week One

Week one has a single focus. I want you to get familiar with the charting system provided and begin the process of tracking your food intake. This week may be frustrating as you start measuring food, planning meals, and calculating nutrients for journaling. The rare person that fails with me fails here. If you're committed to your goals, you'll survive this step and will have virtually guaranteed your success. Take this week very seriously and you'll understand why I feel it's the most critical. Once you go through the learning process of tracking your food, you'll have a literal databank of nutritional information memorized without even trying! As you look up foods, read nutrition fact panels, scour menus, and record your intake, you'll be amazed how easy it becomes.

At the end of the first week, you should be getting into your suggested food ranges consistently. The first couple days will be hit and miss; don't expect yourself to be perfect. The first week is a learning process to help you get used to the documentation and slowly get used to what those suggested protein, carbohydrate, and fat intake ranges mean in terms of real food. It's one thing to see numbers on paper and another to translate them into meals!

Week One Steps to Success:

1) Record your beginning weight, body composition measurements (if you're having a professional monitor body fat percentage), and your suggested nutrient intake totals.

2) Plan a sample day by creating meals that include quality foods as discussed in the book, meal volumes that are appropriate, meal times that fit in your schedule, and adjust the meal amounts until the total amount of protein, carbohydrates, and fat fall into your suggested ranges at the end of the day.

3) Plan ahead for the day and make sure you have the food available that you'll need.

4) Record the food intake throughout the day.

5) Make adjustments for the next day if necessary; remember, this is the first week and you shouldn't be perfect yet!

6) At the end of the week weigh yourself. You will potentially lose a lot of water weight as you use water-holding excess carbs stored in your body.

7) Review your week and focus on "lessons learned" so you can improve for next week.

NUTRITION JOURNAL

DATE: _____ WEEK: _____ DAY: _____ WEIGHT: _____

MEAL	PORTION SIZE	FOOD CONSUMED	TOTAL GRAMS PER MEAL			CALORIES
			Pro	Carb	Fat	
1						
2						
3						
4						
5						
6						
7						
TOTALS FOR DAY						

NUTRITION JOURNAL

DATE: _____ WEEK: _____ DAY: _____ WEIGHT: _____

MEAL	PORTION SIZE	FOOD CONSUMED	TOTAL GRAMS PER MEAL			CALORIES
			Pro	Carb	Fat	
1						
2						
3						
4						
5						
6						
7						
TOTALS FOR DAY						

NUTRITION JOURNAL

DATE: _____ WEEK: _____ DAY: _____ WEIGHT: _____

MEAL	PORTION SIZE	FOOD CONSUMED	TOTAL GRAMS PER MEAL			CALORIES
			Pro	Carb	Fat	
1						
2						
3						
4						
5						
6						
7						
TOTALS FOR DAY						

NUTRITION JOURNAL

DATE: _____   WEEK: _____   DAY: _____   WEIGHT: _____

MEAL	PORTION SIZE	FOOD CONSUMED	TOTAL GRAMS PER MEAL			CALORIES
			Pro	Carb	Fat	
1						
2						
3						
4						
5						
6						
7						
TOTALS FOR DAY						

NUTRITION JOURNAL

DATE: _____   WEEK: _____   DAY: _____   WEIGHT: _____

MEAL	PORTION SIZE	FOOD CONSUMED	TOTAL GRAMS PER MEAL			CALORIES
			Pro	Carb	Fat	
1						
2						
3						
4						
5						
6						
7						
TOTALS FOR DAY						

NUTRITION JOURNAL

DATE: WEEK: DAY: WEIGHT:

MEAL	PORTION SIZE	FOOD CONSUMED	TOTAL GRAMS PER MEAL			CALORIES
			Pro	Carb	Fat	
1						
2						
3						
4						
5						
6						
7						
TOTALS FOR DAY						

NUTRITION JOURNAL

DATE: _____   WEEK: _____   DAY: _____   WEIGHT: _____

MEAL	PORTION SIZE	FOOD CONSUMED	TOTAL GRAMS PER MEAL			CALORIES
			Pro	Carb	Fat	
1						
2						
3						
4						
5						
6						
7						
TOTALS FOR DAY						

Week Two

Hopefully you now agree that going through week one with diligence was critical to your success. Now, you have a great base of experience to know what all those grams of protein, carbohydrates, and fat really mean in a day of food intake. Week two's objective is to refine your meals and work on making sure your program is going to be perfect for you, individually. Chapter Two offered guidance in creating meals that would be fairly consistent in volume, timing, and quality so that the volume of food you start with will be properly consumed throughout the day. Recall that blood chemistry stability is a major factor in how you'll feel and how effective your weight loss will be. I want you to experience more energy than you thought possible and minimize your hunger. This is easily accomplished by focusing on the nuts and bolts of your food throughout the day.

First, this week will be a fair assessment of the amount of food you're consuming. The first week's weight loss was a combination of water loss and fat loss, but this week will allow a better look at actual fat loss. Two-to-three pounds for men and one-to-two pounds for women is about perfect. Faster loss may indicate that you're in danger of losing muscle, getting too hungry, and being prone to overeating when the hunger becomes too great. Review Chapter One on how to adjust your nutrient numbers if you're losing too fast or too slowly.

Glance back through your first week's journal of your food intake. Check for the consistency of your daily numbers, spacing between meals, and meal volume. Are you too high or too low on protein, carbs, or fat? Were there some large gaps between meals (four hours or more)? I disagree with nutritionists that try to get people to have the exact same ratios and amounts of food at exact time intervals, but for all the reasons I discussed Chapter Two, there has to be some consistency. The amount of flexibility I feel is appropriate is for your own hunger patterns and for schedule normalcy. It's common for most people to need more food in the morning and then be less hungry in the after-noon. It can be a scheduling issue as to when you can eat a whole-food meal and when you may need a protein bar or shake. These are elements for you to decide based on your social situation and based on your hunger, likes, and dislikes. If, however, you aren't seeing the results you want, you may have to revisit this step and make sure you're not sabotaging your progress out of convenience. I want to make things as easy as possible, but some aspects may need to be sacrificed for you to progress.

Week Two Steps to Success:

1) Review your first week of journaling. Look at daily nutrient totals, meal spacing, and recall subjective thoughts such as hunger, energy level, and ease of meal consumption.

2) Alter your meal plans if necessary due to schedule inconvenience or hunger patterns. Experiment to see if you can improve for your own comfort level.

3) Purposely alter some meals to increase your variety of foods.

4) Start journaling subjective comments so you can relate your body's response to what you're consuming.

5) Weigh yourself and determine if you're losing too fast or too slow. Adjust your program according to chapter one.

NUTRITION JOURNAL

DATE: _____   WEEK: _____   DAY: _____   WEIGHT: _____

MEAL	PORTION SIZE	FOOD CONSUMED	TOTAL GRAMS PER MEAL			CALORIES
			Pro	Carb	Fat	
1						
2						
3						
4						
5						
6						
7						
TOTALS FOR DAY						

NUTRITION JOURNAL

DATE: _____   WEEK: _____   DAY: _____   WEIGHT: _____

MEAL	PORTION SIZE	FOOD CONSUMED	TOTAL GRAMS PER MEAL			CALORIES
			Pro	Carb	Fat	
1						
2						
3						
4						
5						
6						
7						
		TOTALS FOR DAY				

NUTRITION JOURNAL

DATE: _____ WEEK: _____ DAY: _____ WEIGHT: _____

MEAL	PORTION SIZE	FOOD CONSUMED	TOTAL GRAMS PER MEAL			CALORIES
			Pro	Carb	Fat	
1						
2						
3						
4						
5						
6						
7						
		TOTALS FOR DAY				

NUTRITION JOURNAL

DATE: _____   WEEK: _____   DAY: _____   WEIGHT: _____

MEAL	PORTION SIZE	FOOD CONSUMED	TOTAL GRAMS PER MEAL			CALORIES
			Pro	Carb	Fat	
1						
2						
3						
4						
5						
6						
7						
TOTALS FOR DAY						

NUTRITION JOURNAL

DATE: WEEK: DAY: WEIGHT:

MEAL	PORTION SIZE	FOOD CONSUMED	TOTAL GRAMS PER MEAL			CALORIES
			Pro	Carb	Fat	
1						
2						
3						
4						
5						
6						
7						
TOTALS FOR DAY						

NUTRITION JOURNAL

DATE:　　　　　　WEEK:　　　　　　DAY:　　　　　　WEIGHT:

MEAL	PORTION SIZE	FOOD CONSUMED	TOTAL GRAMS PER MEAL			CALORIES
			Pro	Carb	Fat	
1						
2						
3						
4						
5						
6						
7						
TOTALS FOR DAY						

NUTRITION JOURNAL

DATE: _____ WEEK: _____ DAY: _____ WEIGHT: _____

MEAL	PORTION SIZE	FOOD CONSUMED	Pro	Carb	Fat	CALORIES
1						
2						
3						
4						
5						
6						
7						
		TOTALS FOR DAY				

TOTAL GRAMS PER MEAL

Week Three

Now you're over the hump and on your way to permanent success! Whether you realize it or not, you have altered your eating habits and have gained a great deal of invaluable knowledge by embracing this experience thus far. Those first two weeks constitute the largest "structural" steps in your program. You have fine-tuned your food volume for a typical day that will satisfy proper nutritional needs to lose body fat and maintain or gain lean body mass. If necessary, keep adjusting your totals based on the information in Chapter One if you're losing too fast or too slow. Excellent documentation of your nutrition is key to making sure you have as objective a guide as possible.

It's time to look at the details of the actual food you're consuming. This would be a good time to review Chapter Three and increase your understanding of carbohydrates. The amount of information can be a little overwhelming for some nutritional novices, and success in this area will come from the details. When you're not in a caloric deficit to lose weight, but are maintaining, you'll find you can increase your flexibility and still accomplish your goal. But when you're dieting, the glycemic index, carbohydrate volume per meal, and avoiding sugar and hunger-triggering foods becomes paramount! The closer you stick to the physiological principles in these chapters, the easier it will be for you to succeed!

Carbohydrates, I must repeat, are the body's primary energy source. At this point in your program, you may feel some hunger return if you're generally not eating enough calories. Most people by far feel like they're eating more food than normal just because of the increase in protein, fibrous carbohydrates, and because eating frequently keeps them full. However, it's also a common pattern for people to start letting protein levels slide and start increasing carbohydrate intake again. If you start heading in this direction, it's a slow path back to a plateau. Too much carbohydrate intake will block your body's need to use an alternative energy source, which will be body fat if you keep your carbs in check.

Recall that blood chemistry stability is a great focus. Since carbohydrates will still be where you get most of your blood glucose, you want to make sure you're not elevating it too high at meals or leaving gaping holes in your day without enough. Look at your food journaling and make sure you have some balance in your meals and snacks. They don't have to be exact replicas of each other, but you should avoid too far of a swing up or down in the amount of carbs per meal and still end up with the amount that you have set as a goal. Too many in one meal and you'll end up lethargic and then very hungry. Too few for too many hours and you will also end up hungry and possibly unable to pull the reigns in at the kitchen table.

Week Three Steps to Success:

1) Review chapter three on carbohydrates.

2) Review your daily nutrition intake and take steps to make sure it's consistent daily.

3) Use a good measure of balance in your carbohydrate intake meal-to-meal. Avoid too much in meals and avoid allowing too much time to go by between meals.

4) Start paying close attention to the glycemic index and note which carb sources trigger hunger a short while after the meal and which ones delay hunger.

5) Weigh yourself and adjust your nutrient intake as described in chapter one if necessary.

NUTRITION JOURNAL

DATE: _____ WEEK: _____ DAY: _____ WEIGHT: _____

MEAL	PORTION SIZE	FOOD CONSUMED	TOTAL GRAMS PER MEAL			CALORIES
			Pro	Carb	Fat	
1						
2						
3						
4						
5						
6						
7						
TOTALS FOR DAY						

NUTRITION JOURNAL

DATE: _____ WEEK: _____ DAY: _____ WEIGHT: _____

MEAL	PORTION SIZE	FOOD CONSUMED	Pro	Carb	Fat	CALORIES
1						
2						
3						
4						
5						
6						
7						
		TOTALS FOR DAY				

TOTAL GRAMS PER MEAL

NUTRITION JOURNAL

DATE: WEEK: DAY: WEIGHT:

MEAL	PORTION SIZE	FOOD CONSUMED	TOTAL GRAMS PER MEAL			CALORIES
			Pro	Carb	Fat	
1						
2						
3						
4						
5						
6						
7						
		TOTALS FOR DAY				

NUTRITION JOURNAL

DATE: _____   WEEK: _____   DAY: _____   WEIGHT: _____

MEAL	PORTION SIZE	FOOD CONSUMED	TOTAL GRAMS PER MEAL			CALORIES
			Pro	Carb	Fat	
1						
2						
3						
4						
5						
6						
7						
TOTALS FOR DAY						

NUTRITION JOURNAL

DATE: _____ WEEK: _____ DAY: _____ WEIGHT: _____

MEAL	PORTION SIZE	FOOD CONSUMED	TOTAL GRAMS PER MEAL			CALORIES
			Pro	Carb	Fat	
1						
2						
3						
4						
5						
6						
7						
TOTALS FOR DAY						

NUTRITION JOURNAL

DATE: WEEK: DAY: WEIGHT:

MEAL	PORTION SIZE	FOOD CONSUMED	TOTAL GRAMS PER MEAL			CALORIES
			Pro	Carb	Fat	
1						
2						
3						
4						
5						
6						
7						
TOTALS FOR DAY						

NUTRITION JOURNAL

DATE: _____   WEEK: _____   DAY: _____   WEIGHT: _____

MEAL	PORTION SIZE	FOOD CONSUMED	TOTAL GRAMS PER MEAL			CALORIES
			Pro	Carb	Fat	
1						
2						
3						
4						
5						
6						
7						
TOTALS FOR DAY						

Week Four

I like to view fat as a variable second to carbohydrates that can be used to sustain body fat loss if manipulated correctly. Chapter Four provides plenty of detail regarding the function of fat in the body and the differences between "good" and "bad" fat. The practical application of fat can be simplified. Once you have created some good habits, including the addition of some healthy unsaturated and perhaps "medicinal" fats, you'll have to cut the saturated fats to a minimum to stay within your daily range. If fat intake is as moderate as I suggest and healthy fats are the dominant source, then dietary fat will never take the blame for lack of progress. However, if the table starts tilting toward an increased fat intake (especially with a higher inclusion of saturated fats), a cascade of events will take place. First, the calorie-rich fat may take you right up to a maintenance range of food intake from your planned calorie deficit. This is common in people that mistakenly think carbs are the only thing to worry about. A hefty handful of almonds may seem like the best thing to eat to avoid letting the carbs get too high, but if the extra fat increases the total calories for the day out of a deficit range, a day of fat loss is missed.

Second, fat can be absorbed straight from the bloodstream and into your fat cells. Too much fat in a meal on a day in which calories weren't low enough and you may go beyond a lost day of progress and actually regain a small amount of fat. Excessive amounts of fat can only be used as energy successfully if carbs are near zero, such as in a ketogenic diet. As previously discussed, however, this isn't the best or easiest way to lose weight. Make sure you're not letting your fat creep up if you tend to focus primarily on carbs.

The bottom line is to make sure you include a variety of healthy unsaturated fats wherever you can in your diet. Allow the balance to be made up from foods you like and include in your weekly plan. Keep fat sources spaced fairly evenly throughout the day and it will be easier to stay in your suggested ranges, for it will help slow digestion, maintain blood glucose levels, and keep hunger in check.

Week Four Steps to Success:

1) Pick a variety of unsaturated fats that can be used as at least 50% of your fat intake

2) Space fat intake as evenly as possible within meal structure.

3) Don't let fat intake creep up just to keep carbs down.

4) Perform your weekly review of nutrition journaling for consistency and check your body weight for progress. Make your best effort to correct problem areas in carrying out your program and adjust your program according to chapter one if necessary.

NUTRITION JOURNAL

DATE: _____   WEEK: _____   DAY: _____   WEIGHT: _____

MEAL	PORTION SIZE	FOOD CONSUMED	TOTAL GRAMS PER MEAL			CALORIES
			Pro	Carb	Fat	
1						
2						
3						
4						
5						
6						
7						
TOTALS FOR DAY						

NUTRITION JOURNAL

DATE: _____ WEEK: _____ DAY: _____ WEIGHT: _____

MEAL	PORTION SIZE	FOOD CONSUMED	TOTAL GRAMS PER MEAL			CALORIES
			Pro	Carb	Fat	
1						
2						
3						
4						
5						
6						
7						
TOTALS FOR DAY						

NUTRITION JOURNAL

DATE:_____   WEEK:_____   DAY:_____   WEIGHT:_____

MEAL	PORTION SIZE	FOOD CONSUMED	TOTAL GRAMS PER MEAL			CALORIES
			Pro	Carb	Fat	
1						
2						
3						
4						
5						
6						
7						
		TOTALS FOR DAY				

NUTRITION JOURNAL

DATE: _____   WEEK: _____   DAY: _____   WEIGHT: _____

MEAL	PORTION SIZE	FOOD CONSUMED	TOTAL GRAMS PER MEAL			CALORIES
			Pro	Carb	Fat	
1						
2						
3						
4						
5						
6						
7						
TOTALS FOR DAY						

NUTRITION JOURNAL

DATE: WEEK: DAY: WEIGHT:

MEAL	PORTION SIZE	FOOD CONSUMED	TOTAL GRAMS PER MEAL			CALORIES
			Pro	Carb	Fat	
1						
2						
3						
4						
5						
6						
7						
TOTALS FOR DAY						

NUTRITION JOURNAL

DATE: _____ WEEK: _____ DAY: _____ WEIGHT: _____

MEAL	PORTION SIZE	FOOD CONSUMED	TOTAL GRAMS PER MEAL			CALORIES
			Pro	Carb	Fat	
1						
2						
3						
4						
5						
6						
7						
		TOTALS FOR DAY				

NUTRITION JOURNAL

DATE: _____   WEEK: _____   DAY: _____   WEIGHT: _____

MEAL	PORTION SIZE	FOOD CONSUMED	TOTAL GRAMS PER MEAL			CALORIES
			Pro	Carb	Fat	
1						
2						
3						
4						
5						
6						
7						
TOTALS FOR DAY						

Week Five

Protein is included last among the three macronutrients due to its lesser direct role in fat loss, but to minimize its role would be a mistake. As a matter of fact, I find that behaviorally it is one of the best indicators of a client's success. I won't repeat the body's need for and use of amino acids for cell function; I'll stick to what will help you lose and control weight permanently. Most who embark upon this journey with me will have to raise their protein to a level they're not used to. I certainly don't advocate an unsafe, unhealthy, or even unnecessary level of protein intake, but most of us just don't eat enough. That's a controversial statement since we can survive on very little, but I'm after thriving, not surviving.

When protein is consumed, it is digested slowly. Other foods eaten at the same time are therefore digested and absorbed slowly as well. After those meals, blood chemistry will be more stable for a longer period. Hunger will be lower and energy will be higher. You don't have to eat protein at every meal, but there are some key meals. Breakfast is a good place to eat some protein to prevent hunger shortly thereafter. If you can't eat much protein after breakfast, make sure you get some in your first snack; maybe a protein bar or shake. Supper is also a meal in which you want to have a whole food protein source to help prevent late evening hunger. My suggestions are based on what can help you succeed due to years of experience, but should be coupled with your own personal observations of your hunger patterns and schedule preferences.

The practical side of protein that I mentioned in the first paragraph relates heavily to hunger. It is so common a pattern that I don't want you to overlook the possibility in your eating. It may have taken you a week or two to get your protein levels up to your suggested ranges. While weight loss is steady and energy is increasing, it is easy to ride this high just because of the positive reinforcement. But eventually, the rigors of daily life start competing with that momentum and it's easier to make choices due to convenience instead of conviction. Protein intake starts decreasing, hunger therefore increases, and reflexively, carbohydrate consumption increases again. Voila: the recipe for slipping out of a body fat burning mode.

Week Five Steps to Success:

1) Make sure protein levels aren't sliding downward.

2) Keep protein levels lean whenever possible. Save fattier sources for occasional meals.

3) Consider protein bars or shakes for snacks if protein levels are difficult to achieve.

4) Review your charting and look for a link between lower protein days and increased hunger and possible increases in carb intake.

5) Review charting and look for a link between unwanted hunger and lower protein meals preceding the hunger. Consider increasing protein at those meals.

6) Check body weight for progress and adjust nutrient numbers per chapter one if necessary.

NUTRITION JOURNAL

DATE: _____ WEEK: _____ DAY: _____ WEIGHT: _____

MEAL	PORTION SIZE	FOOD CONSUMED	TOTAL GRAMS PER MEAL			CALORIES
			Pro	Carb	Fat	
1						
2						
3						
4						
5						
6						
7						
		TOTALS FOR DAY				

		NUTRITION JOURNAL				

DATE: _____   WEEK: _____   DAY: _____   WEIGHT: _____

MEAL	PORTION SIZE	FOOD CONSUMED	TOTAL GRAMS PER MEAL			CALORIES
			Pro	Carb	Fat	
1						
2						
3						
4						
5						
6						
7						
TOTALS FOR DAY						

NUTRITION JOURNAL

DATE: _____ WEEK: _____ DAY: _____ WEIGHT: _____

MEAL	PORTION SIZE	FOOD CONSUMED	TOTAL GRAMS PER MEAL			CALORIES
			Pro	Carb	Fat	
1						
2						
3						
4						
5						
6						
7						
TOTALS FOR DAY						

NUTRITION JOURNAL

DATE: _____ WEEK: _____ DAY: _____ WEIGHT: _____

MEAL	PORTION SIZE	FOOD CONSUMED	TOTAL GRAMS PER MEAL			CALORIES
			Pro	Carb	Fat	
1						
2						
3						
4						
5						
6						
7						
		TOTALS FOR DAY				

NUTRITION JOURNAL

DATE: _____ WEEK: _____ DAY: _____ WEIGHT: _____

MEAL	PORTION SIZE	FOOD CONSUMED	TOTAL GRAMS PER MEAL			CALORIES
			Pro	Carb	Fat	
1						
2						
3						
4						
5						
6						
7						
		TOTALS FOR DAY				

NUTRITION JOURNAL

DATE: _____   WEEK: _____   DAY: _____   WEIGHT: _____

MEAL	PORTION SIZE	FOOD CONSUMED	TOTAL GRAMS PER MEAL			CALORIES
			Pro	Carb	Fat	
1						
2						
3						
4						
5						
6						
7						
		TOTALS FOR DAY				

NUTRITION JOURNAL

DATE: _____   WEEK: _____   DAY: _____   WEIGHT: _____

MEAL	PORTION SIZE	FOOD CONSUMED	TOTAL GRAMS PER MEAL			CALORIES
			Pro	Carb	Fat	
1						
2						
3						
4						
5						
6						
7						
TOTALS FOR DAY						

Week Six

You're now coasting into or through the middle portion of your weight loss program. Reviewing all the key points in this six-week program from time-to-time will help keep the driving principles in the forefront of your mind. You may also consider reading certain chapters again for additional assessment of your progress. Week six is dedicated to an evaluation of your progress and a management plan for the rest of your time in weight-loss mode. After that, you'll reach the incredible day of being able to celebrate the success of reaching your goal and increasing your food toward maintenance levels!

Before we get there, however, let's keep our hands on the plow and make sure we have the good fortune of reaching that point. Look at your daily charting of protein, carbohydrate, and fat intake. Carefully compare that information to your weight loss progress. Pay attention even to overall calorie intake. Calculate weekly averages for those statistics and look for the relationship between the level of food and macronutrients you're eating and your rate of weight loss. You should be able to see a causal relationship between the two. You can observe with clarity and precision how much food you can eat each day (on average) and lose one pound, two pounds, or whatever your rate, based on these records. Now you may see one reason I dictate that this documentation is key to your success. You have created a literal database that will enable you to manage your weight control for as long as you wish.

That is exactly our goal for the remainder of your program. Decide what pace you would like to continue at (based on my recommendations of safe weight loss and your own comfort level) and plan meals and daily nutritional totals accordingly. Keep monitoring your progress and recording your food intake as you add to your database. Understand that there will be an occasional setback or a social situation at which you plan to not "eat perfectly" according to your plan, but if these are infrequent, you'll see your progress continue.

Week Six Steps to Success:

1) Review weekly weight loss rate and compare with weekly averages of all three macronutrients.

2) Compare the relationship of this data for accurate estimations of the food intake required for different rates of weekly weight loss.

3) Celebrate the completion of your first six weeks!!

NUTRITION JOURNAL

DATE:_____ WEEK:_____ DAY:_____ WEIGHT:_____

MEAL	PORTION SIZE	FOOD CONSUMED	TOTAL GRAMS PER MEAL			CALORIES
			Pro	Carb	Fat	
1						
2						
3						
4						
5						
6						
7						
TOTALS FOR DAY						

NUTRITION JOURNAL

DATE: _____ WEEK: _____ DAY: _____ WEIGHT: _____

MEAL	PORTION SIZE	FOOD CONSUMED	TOTAL GRAMS PER MEAL			CALORIES
			Pro	Carb	Fat	
1						
2						
3						
4						
5						
6						
7						
TOTALS FOR DAY						

NUTRITION JOURNAL

DATE: _____   WEEK: _____   DAY: _____   WEIGHT: _____

MEAL	PORTION SIZE	FOOD CONSUMED	TOTAL GRAMS PER MEAL			CALORIES
			Pro	Carb	Fat	
1						
2						
3						
4						
5						
6						
7						
TOTALS FOR DAY						

NUTRITION JOURNAL

DATE: _____ WEEK: _____ DAY: _____ WEIGHT: _____

MEAL	PORTION SIZE	FOOD CONSUMED	TOTAL GRAMS PER MEAL			CALORIES
			Pro	Carb	Fat	
1						
2						
3						
4						
5						
6						
7						
TOTALS FOR DAY						

NUTRITION JOURNAL

DATE: _____ WEEK: _____ DAY: _____ WEIGHT: _____

MEAL	PORTION SIZE	FOOD CONSUMED	TOTAL GRAMS PER MEAL			CALORIES
			Pro	Carb	Fat	
1						
2						
3						
4						
5						
6						
7						
TOTALS FOR DAY						

NUTRITION JOURNAL

DATE: _____ WEEK: _____ DAY: _____ WEIGHT: _____

MEAL	PORTION SIZE	FOOD CONSUMED	TOTAL GRAMS PER MEAL			CALORIES
			Pro	Carb	Fat	
1						
2						
3						
4						
5						
6						
7						
TOTALS FOR DAY						

NUTRITION JOURNAL

DATE: WEEK: DAY: WEIGHT:

MEAL	PORTION SIZE	FOOD CONSUMED	TOTAL GRAMS PER MEAL			CALORIES
			Pro	Carb	Fat	
1						
2						
3						
4						
5						
6						
7						
		TOTALS FOR DAY				

Monthly Nutrition Log

Week One

Day	Protein	Carbs	Fat	Calories	Comments	Weight
1						
2						
3						
4						
5						
6						
7						
Averages						

Week Two

Day	Protein	Carbs	Fat	Calories	Comments	Weight
1						
2						
3						
4						
5						
6						
7						
Averages						

Week Three

Day	Protein	Carbs	Fat	Calories	Comments	Weight
1						
2						
3						
4						
5						
6						
7						
Averages						

Monthly Nutrition Log

Day	Protein	Carbs	Fat	Calories	Comments	Weight
Week Four						
1						
2						
3						
4						
5						
6						
7						
Averages						

Day	Protein	Carbs	Fat	Calories	Comments	Weight
Week Five						
1						
2						
3						
4						
5						
6						
7						
Averages						

Day	Protein	Carbs	Fat	Calories	Comments	Weight
Week Six						
1						
2						
3						
4						
5						
6						
7						
Averages						

10

SUCCESSFULLY PROGRESSING TO MAINTENANCE

There would be nothing more disheartening than to gain back a significant portion of the weight you lost once you've worked so hard for so long. You may already know exactly what I'm talking about from past experience. This need not be a pattern if you pay attention to this chapter.

Some of the blame for this misfortune lies, again, at the foot of physiology. The habits created when dieting and the excitement of success held you to your previous plan. However, if that plan included a severe decrease in carbohydrates or insufficient calories, your metabolic rate may have suffered significantly. Once a higher food intake is reestablished, you may have stored body fat rapidly until your metabolic rate rebounded. By then, it was too late. That is the danger of not keeping sufficient calories, especially in the form of protein and carbohydrates, in your diet.

A second reason for failure, and often in conjunction with the first, is letting your guard down and not adjusting your food properly. If you were to hit a few days of really high carb intake, especially the typical binge or "celebration"-type foods, it is very hard to recover. The wildly fluctuating blood sugar levels will spin you into levels of hunger you aren't used to. Before you know it, you're eating an incredible amount of carbohydrates and converting a large portion of them into body fat again. This is the exact cycle you bought this book to avoid. Here's how:

Once you have reached your goal, you have to bring your food intake up to a maintenance level where you will no longer be losing, but, of course, not gaining. You will not have to raise your protein levels, for they have already been set to give you an ideal amount. Your fat and carbohydrates may be raised in tandem but not necessarily in equal amounts. You may find that 10 to 15 extra grams of fat and 25 grams of carbs provided enough energy and calories to be the first step toward raising your food intake up to a maintenance level. This may slow your rate of loss, but not stop it completely. Take another step upward, and then another. Many important things will happen if you make this process incremental. First, your blood chemistry will remain more stable and you'll be less likely to experience binge-causing hunger due to the increase in carbohydrates. Second, you'll slowly rebuild any decreases in your metabolic rate that may have occurred due to the length of your diet. This will ensure that you won't regain body fat at all. As a matter of fact, you'll find you have to slowly keep adding more food to not lose weight! The amount of carbohydrates and fat that you add is entirely up to you, but keep several health and behavioral points in mind.

You still want to adhere to the same health-building habits that you created along the way. Keep good fats in your diet and keep saturated fats low. Stick with low-glycemic index carbs as much as you can (for all the reasons you dieted with them). If you can maintain most of these principles, your increase in food will leave you with high energy, stability, and controlled weight. Experiment with different levels of carbohydrates and fat at your decided maintenance level of food. You may find that you feel better and "operate" better with one having been raised disproportionately to the other. This has to do with metabolic body type. An insulin-sensitive person may get hungrier on a higher level of carbs and tend to gain weight back. However, with carbs remaining a little lower and fat increasing, the same person may have no hunger, high energy, and no weight gain. A person fortunate enough to have a high metabolism tends to be an "ectomorph" and be able to consume a higher percentage of calories from carbs without weight gain. Beware, though, for despite being able to get away with more carbs, an ectomorph can still gain weight.

One last point: As you transition into maintenance, you are going from a dieting level of food that includes less carbs than your body needs for energy. This, of course, is why you're body is converting body fat into glucose and you're losing weight. As you increase your food, however, you will be refilling your liver and muscles with a higher amount of glycogen. Glycogen attracts and holds water. You will undoubtedly gain a couple of pounds of water (just as your first couple of lost pounds were water). Don't be alarmed; this is normal hydration and a normal level of carbohydrates stored in your body. You just want to make sure you don't gain more than a couple pounds back once you've hit your lowest weight. Your body fat level won't be affected; the weight will be just water and glycogen. This is another reason to keep your upward changes slow and incremental. You don't want to fret over water gain, but you also don't want to be self-deceived into thinking that you're gaining just water when it may be fat.

So, there you have it. If patiently and scientifically handled, the transition into maintenance can be smooth and successful. Instead of regain, you can have an increasing level of energy, an increasing metabolic rate, and control of your weight. That, after all, is my goal for you.

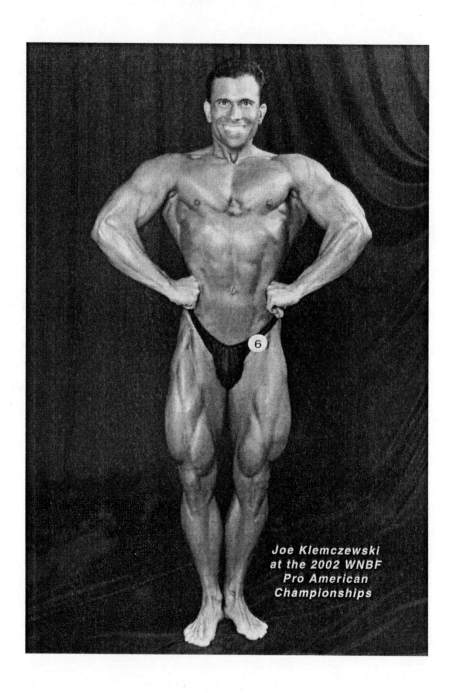

*Joe Klemczewski
at the 2002 WNBF
Pro American
Championships*

APPENDIX

BODYBUILDERS AND OTHER PHYSIQUE EXTREMISTS

There exist among us those that aren't satisfied with normal levels of success. Call them Type A personalities, overachievers, or insanely obsessive-compulsive, but they're all the same. Tell them that 10 percent body fat is a healthy and admirable goal, and they want five percent. For some bodybuilders, athletes, and others with physique-dependent careers, one has to go beyond "normal" nutrition. You may want to go farther than your body is used to and push against metabolic set-point barriers. This special chapter is for these "extreme" dieting cases, but its tips and advice will be useful to every reader.

The Motivation

It is often easier to achieve extreme results than good results. Those with a physique-dependent goal such as competing in a bodybuilding contest have a greater sense of accountability because there's a time limit and a competitive agenda. External motivation is a great tool that can spur even the tame towards unexpected success. If there is an event you are preparing for, create a comprehensive plan. Record where you are now and where you want to be. Fill in the gap with incremental checkpoints so you can monitor your progress. Some like to stay motivated with pictures, positive slogans, and reminders pinned up at home, work, and on the refrigerator.

Metabolic Transformation in Action

"As with most things in life, you reach many plateaus while striving for your goals. I had reached the height of my natural bodybuilding career by finally becoming a professional after many years of training. The major challenge I faced while preparing for a contest was that of "peaking" correctly. By this, I mean being at my leanest, lowest body fat levels and eating and training at exactly the levels which would enable me to look my best the day of the contest. I already know I could get very lean but to feel physically and mentally good leading up to the show has been my main challenge. My goal is to "enjoy the ride" as I prepare for competition but it is hard to do when you don't feel mentally energetic or positive.

For the first time in my career I did step on stage looking my best and also feeling my best ever! I owe this all to Dr. Joe who has been my nutrition coach and motivator through my journey of winning the heavyweight title at the Ms. International. Joe took all the stress and questioning from me and gave me nutrition goals for each month, week, and day! Because he competes at the professional level he knows what has to be done and what it takes. I never felt deprived or tired with Joe's suggestions and best of all, I felt stronger than ever while competing (as he said would happen if I followed his instructions!) Dr. Joe has such great communication skills, patience, and dedication to his clients. He has successfully helped me reach my goal!"

photo by Sandra Lynch

Karen Miller, WNBF Ms. Universe & Ms. International

Individual Approaches

When you decide it's time to start dieting, where do you begin? If you're like me, it will be with protein. How much protein do you need to build, or more appropriately, maintain your muscle mass? For a bodybuilder, I would always start with a base of at least one gram of protein per pound of lean body mass. I like to add a little buffer because of additional cardio and to guard against inadvertent catabolism. I add even more if a client is an ectomorph that loses weight easily. As that person gets closer to a contest, if he/she is on track to be ready ahead of schedule (my typical plan), then I add even more. For example, I have one client that is a WNBF title-holder, is currently six weeks away from a contest, and meets every one of the criteria for adding protein. He is currently carrying several more pounds of muscle than he had at last year's contest, and is consuming more than two grams of protein per pound of lean body mass! Keep in mind that this is an ectomorph with a high metabolism battling to maintain muscle. Not everyone would ever need or even be able to use that much protein.

Protein intake should match your requirements as a bodybuilder, but not necessarily at the expense of other important nutrients. The client I mentioned above is also consuming 250 grams of carbs per day. I haven't raised his protein exponentially at the cost of muscle-sparing, energy-building carbohydrates, or fat. These two nutrients are where most of us are a little confused. Should I eat no carbs, low carbs, or moderate carbs? And what about fat? Should I eat some red meat, or maybe just flaxseed oil, or maybe no fat at all? I get emails all the time that begin with, "I heard this..." and end with, "...is that true?" Here's where you need to really pay attention.

Your body type will give you a great starting point in determining what type of dieting is best for you. To determine whether you'll be more effective with a higher or lower carbohydrate diet, you have to decide if you're an ectomorph that has a very hard time gaining weight, a mesomorph who can gain weight and has a decent muscular frame, or an endomorph that gains weight very easily. You can also characterize yourself in different degrees, such as an extreme ectomorph that has a very light muscular frame and can barely gain five pounds in the off season. Or maybe you're a moderate endomorph that has a lot of muscle, can gain weight easily, but doesn't have a terrible time losing when you need to. Recall that carbohydrates are the most muscle-sparing nutrient we eat. More so than protein, carbs will buffer against muscle loss. I always want my clients to eat as many carbs as they can and still lose weight. Due to differences in body type, that may be a gigantic difference for two clients of the same size, but I still want as many as possible.

An ectomorph is generally very efficient at glucose metabolism. Ectomorphs don't convert a lot of excess glucose into body fat because they use it rapidly for energy. This person needs more carbs more frequently to maintain muscle mass and energy. Making up for it in protein and fat isn't as effective as a higher amount of carb intake if their protein and fat is already adequate.

Slow metabolic endomorphs do much better with a lower amount of carbs. If this person consumes too many carbs throughout the day, then glucose metabolism (which is a slower process for an endomorph) blocks ketogenic metabolism, where body fat can be used for energy. Remember that when you have carbs that are available to be used as energy, they will be. If your body is slow at using carbs, as indicated by a slower metabolic rate and carbs making you look "soft," then you have to eat a low enough amount so that your body will turn to its stored fat for energy. I still like to keep carbs as high as possible for this type of client, but for the slowest of the slow (metabolically) brief spurts of very low-carb dieting are sometimes required.

An easy way to give yourself a solid starting point is to set your protein intake first. Determine how many calories you think you need to reach your goals. Next, add about 20-25 percent of your total calories from fat. Then, fill in the rest with carbs. Track your nutrition meticulously for two weeks, and take notes on how you feel and how your workouts are going. If progress is too slow or too rapid, analyze your plan in light of your body type. Are you too high or too low on protein? Adjust your carbs up or down as needed. You can also adjust your fat. I rarely go below 15 percent on fat intake, but I also don't like to go too high. Once you get above 25 percent of your total calories from fat, you could use those extra calories as protein or carbs for a greater benefit than the additional fat can give.

Metabolic Transformation in Action

"I have been competing for more than five years and have read and covered every possible way to compete and try to win my weight class. A lot of advice came from the magazines and seemed to leave me just short of taking home that first place trophy. I wanted to make it without help from anyone and my stubbornness got in the way.

During the past year I finally finished six years of working and going to school full time and completed my Certified Strength and Conditioning Specialist certification through the NSCA. Things would be easier now, so I thought. In the beginning of 2002 I was on a mission to win my first bodybuilding show. After taking the first ten weeks of preparation on my own, I finally decided to get help from a professional. I really researched to find someone who had the credentials and ran across an article by Dr. Joe Klemczewski in Natural Bodybuilding & Fitness magazine. The first thing I did was order his book to get a feel for his ideas. I knew this was what I needed; it was going to take me to the next level. I made the decision to hire Joe with about six weeks left. Time was not on my side. Joe told me not to panic, but my road was going to be tough. I was ready for the challenge.

Joe looked at my pictures and current body composition statistics. He could see the genetic potential and gave me the initial breakdown of my program. I emailed him my daily journals which he used together with my body comp measurements as we moved forward. My tightness and shape were far better than any previous years. I won the bantamweight classes in two shows. Judges who had seen me before were so impressed with the changes that I was called "the most improved bodybuilder" by a magazine staff writer and was noted as having "defined hamstrings, massive quads, ripped abs, and popping biceps." Part of what made this possible is the last critical week before the contest. Dr. Joe calls it "Peak Week" and I can't thank him enough for essentially laying out every last detail. It was the last piece of the puzzle that can be the most important for anyone entering a bodybuilding show.

Dr. Joe has reestablished my goals and I have one more obstacle to overcome. That goal is to win my pro card and I will definitely have Joe in my corner."

Craig Yarnall, INBF Bodybuilder

I realize this raises as many questions as it answers. The adjusting and monitoring of a specific person's nutrition—and determining if it's the absolute best way of dieting—is very much an individual process, even amid so many scientific constants. The true art of this process lies in using all the science available and molding it to a single person. Whether I work with a WNBF world champion or a 55-year-old heart attack survivor, the program becomes a process. Constant tracking, monitoring, adjusting, and analyzing, shapes the program into what works perfectly for that person. I suggest no less for you. Start now. Create an initial program. Track it flawlessly. Make adjustments one at a time so you can monitor your body's reaction, and don't be afraid to keep trying new things until you're confident you know how your body responds best. You may just stumble upon perfection!

Protein Revisited

Nutritionally speaking, protein is obviously a large part of muscle growth. Protein is made up of amino acids, and amino acids are stored in muscle tissue, stimulate muscle tissue growth, and repair muscle tissue. I'm sure this isn't news to anyone reading this section. However, there are several principles of protein utilization that you may need to work harder on. Collectively, they will give you results proportional to your consistency in following them. In order of importance, the principles are:

1. Volume of protein

2. Frequency of protein

3. Protein quality

4. Amino acid utilization

5. Consistency

Volume of protein is the first step that you must establish in creating the best environment for muscle growth. Remember that protein is broken down into amino acids, which are the keys to repair and growth. By order of your brain, a specific level of amino acids should be circulating in your blood at all times. Even though muscle growth may be your biggest goal in life, your brain needs amino acids for the millions of chemical reactions taking place in your body at every second! If there is a shortage in your bloodstream, your brain simply harvests more from "storage." Your liver stores a short supply for second-by-second needs, but the mother-lode storage site is your muscle tissue. So, every time your bloodstream is low in amino acids, more hard-earned muscle goes down the drain! This is what is coined as a "negative nitrogen balance." Amino acids are nitrogen compounds. Eating enough protein per day is essential for providing these amino acids from your diet instead of your delts. So, simply stated, your muscles will receive the amino acids they need to recover, but it's up to you to either supply them from food or let them be taken from muscle somewhere else in your body.

How much protein is required per day? This is a question I explored for my Master's Thesis. I found it to be controversial when you look at extremes. A vegetarian that claims you can live on 30 grams a day is correct. A bicep-bigger-than-brain gym thug that says 500 grams a day won't kill you is also correct. If you are not active, not seeking to gain muscle, and don't mind your body having very little muscle holding your skeleton together, then eat 30-50 grams a day. If you want to convert extra protein into body fat, stress your kidneys, and create an acidic body pH (good for disease and illness) then I suggest over 500 grams a day. If you are active, seeking muscle, training hard, drink plenty of water, and want the best recovery, then I would go with 1-1.25 grams of protein per pound of lean body mass per day. For example, if I weigh 200 pounds at 10 percent body fat, then my lean body mass is 180 pounds. I would therefore eat 180-225 grams of protein per day. If you are dieting and perhaps hitting cardio aggressively, you may want to jump up to 1-1.5 grams per pound of lean body mass to make sure you're sparing muscle from being used as energy. If you have any general health, liver, or renal conditions, your physician should be consulted before you make any changes to your nutrition. These suggestions, however, are very safe and effective for keeping amino acid levels from dipping for long periods of time.

Frequency of protein consumed throughout the day is closely associated with the overall amount you eat per day. Every time you eat protein, your stomach digests it into amino acids that are released into your small intestine for absorption. Blood levels of amino acids start rising, allowing your recovering muscles to use them for repair and growth without having to harvest them from other areas of your body. Once that protein is digested and absorbed, blood levels of amino acids start leveling off and can get too low (negative nitrogen balance)—unless you eat protein again. If you don't, your body simply starts stripping other muscles to "feed" the muscles that need the nutritional support (the ones most recently worked). This robbing-Peter-to-pay-Paul scenario occurs in more hard-training people than you can imagine. I believe it's the Number One reason that most people don't ever reach their full genetic potential. Amino acids are simply shifted around the body from workout to workout. Staying in a positive nitrogen balance requires eating enough protein per day, but it also requires eating protein consistently throughout the day.

The common solution is to eat every three hours. This certainly eliminates a great deal of "dead space" when your body is going without dietary protein, but it can be improved even more by addressing the quality of protein in your diet.

Quality of protein takes over where frequency leaves off. There are a handful of rating systems that attempt to tell us the value of the protein we eat. Most still use the Biological Value Scale (BV), though the Protein Digestibility Corrective Amino Acid Scale (PDCAAS) is the latest and probably most complete. These scales simply tell us how much of the protein is going to be used by our bodies. Meat sources rank the lowest because the digestibility of the protein from the meat fiber (animal muscle) isn't as complete as something like whey isolate. The isolate is processed, removing things like lactose, leaving a more pure source of protein with a lower molecular weight. It's easier to break down and more of it gets absorbed.

The molecular weight of the protein dictates how long digestion has to occur before the amino acids can be used, and to some extent how much will actually get absorbed. Another key to protein quality, however, is the type of amino acids that are in the protein source. Almost every protein imaginable has pros and cons. One protein source may be high in some amino acids but lower in others as compared to another source. It is a very good idea to get your protein from a variety of sources. If you want to go a step further, I would even recommend alternating whole food and engineered food meals. Whole food protein takes longer to digest, tends to fill you up due to its sheer bulk, and allows you to craft other good whole foods into the meal (carbs, fat, fiber, etc.). Consuming a protein shake or bar between whole food meals is more convenient, and you get the benefit of that particular protein source on a scheduled basis. Due to digestive physiology, it's more efficient to alternate meals in this manner, and the net result is more time in a positive nitrogen balance.

Amino acid utilization has a lot to do with protein quality and, as you've already learned, protein frequency. To review: Getting protein into your body at regular intervals is critical to keeping amino acids available for your recovering muscles around the clock. But remember that different protein sources contain different amino acid profiles. Most of us have chicken, turkey, fish, and some red meat as our protein staples. We also choose from the same supplemental protein sources available on the shelves of our gym pro shops or health food stores. My goal would be that you become as educated as possible and learn to separate marketing hype from true ingredient quality. Some very inferior protein products are bestsellers in the industry due to overwhelming self-promotion.

Metabolic Transformation in Action

"I started working with Dr. Joe this past spring about three weeks before competing in Nancy Andrew's INBF Northeast Classic. I felt that I was fairly lean, but since my objective this time out was to earn my pro card I didn't want to leave the peaking process to chance. I had to come in on the day of the show in my best shape ever.

I competed in my first bodybuilding show in 1986. Achieving leanness has never been terribly difficult for me, but peak week has always been a bit of a mystery. My pre-contest insanity would complicate matters by compelling me to scramble that last week desperately searching for the perfect strategy to time things just right. I would try all sorts of crazy dietary tricks to come in full, yet bone-dry, the day of the show. Sometimes it worked and sometimes it didn't. The only consistent outcome was the fact that I would feel pretty sick. Well, not this time. I was leaving nothing to chance.

Joe provided me with very precise instructions as to what my food intake should be. He would assess my progress through our daily email communication and make adjustments accordingly. I came in harder and more vascular than I ever had before. I won the show and my pro card. I continued to work with Joe and went on a month later to win my first pro show, the WNBF Universe.

My challenge, going forward, is to add a little more muscle to my ectomorphic frame. Joe, of course, is helping me accomplish this. We're monitoring my diet and making sure that I get plenty of rest between heavy training sessions. Wish me luck! I'll see you in November 2003 at the WNBF World Championships."

Jody Poirier, Ms. Universe

My work in the study of protein blends is based on the fact that different protein sources have different amino acid profiles and molecular weights. This affects how fast or slow the amino acids leave the stomach and enter the small intestine for absorption. In essence, the gastric emptying intervals can create a functional "time-released" buffet of amino acids for your muscles to draw upon. This type of protein is great between solid meals, but I would also recommend using some pure isolates surrounding your workouts. The cross-flow micro filtered (CFM) and enzyme hydrolyzed are the highest quality isolates you can use (due to the least amount of adulteration during processing).

To tightly summarize every step: Start with the right volume of protein for a day. Next, break that protein intake into evenly spaced, frequent meals. Alternate and vary the type of protein sources to vary the amino acid content. Include high-quality supplemented protein because of its high biological value rating. Starting big and working down through the details is all aimed towards keeping amino acids flowing into your bloodstream as continuously as possible. Staying in this positive nitrogen balance will ensure maximal results.

Consistency with this type of nutritional detail management is what will pay off big time. If you pay this much attention to your nutrition only part-time, you'll get part-time results. If you do it as perfectly as you can, then at the end of this year you may have spent 20 percent more time in a positive nitrogen balance then last year. Maybe 50 percent! Would you take a 20 percent increase in potential muscle gain? How about adding that up for the next five years; what would you look like then? Sow with massive effort and you'll reap massive rewards.

The Role of Carbs

Let's start with your beginning condition. If you're a rookie to competition, you may not have learned that the harder and longer you have to diet, the more muscle you'll lose. The 1960s and 1970s off season approach of pizza, beer, and 70 pounds certainly makes the bench press more impressive, and your mass increases dramatically. That is until reality sets in and you have to lose five pounds a week to fit into your posing trunks. As your body weight and lean body mass increases, so does your body fat. Over-consumption is the quickest way to gain muscle...and fat. The problem is, dieting is the fastest way to lose both as well. I believe going through a couple of serious weight-gaining periods when you're new to training is essential to pack on your genetic potential for muscle, but doing it every year will only hurt your chances of winning. Once you've gained as much muscle as you can, it's not a matter of how much you gain in the off season, it's how much you keep in the pre-contest season. The slower you can lose body fat, the more muscle you'll retain. I like clients to only have to lose a pound or less per week. That means your off season has to be very, very effective in terms of gaining muscle without too much fat.

Despite the great importance of protein, excess protein can be used as energy or converted to body fat. Using protein as energy means less body fat is being used as energy. So, having the right amount of protein plus a little extra "just to be sure" you have enough is optimal, but gross overages of protein aren't going to help you build muscle or retain it.

Believe it or not, carbs are key to retaining muscle. Carbohydrates and insulin have been targeted as the deadly duo in obesity and weight loss for very good reasons. However, even though excess carbs will make you gain fat fast, the silver lining is that you gain and retain muscle through the same mechanism. Even when dieting with a lower-than-normal carb intake, your carbs can be targeted to help you retain muscle, maintain energy levels, and keep your metabolic rate high. The anabolic effects of carbohydrates have been well-documented since a 1940s study showed them to be "protein sparing." Compared to a fasting group, those with carbs (still no protein) lost only half as much muscle as those without carbs. Throw protein in and you get the same effect, just at a higher level. Those with less carbs lose more muscle. Protein is certainly still king in the body's anti-catabolism campaign, but carbohydrates are just as important.

The real trick is in the numbers and, as I mentioned, in the timing. Since you have to limit your body's primary source of energy, carbohydrates, to lose fat, and you want as much glucose as possible to spare muscle, where's the fine line? Once your protein intake is where it should be—high enough to retain muscle but not so high as to cause body fat conversion—then we can look at fat. Fat and carbs go hand-in-hand while dieting. Your body is typically dominant in one of two types of calorie burning at a time. Both are always happening, but one is much higher at given times. They are glucose metabolism and keto-genic metabolism. Your body is either using glucose (carbs) or fat (dietary and stored) for energy. I recommend keeping dietary fat at 15-20 percent of calorie intake while dieting, and then dropping a little lower as the show draws near. This enables you to eat more muscle-sparing carbs. The more you restrict carb intake, the more time you spend burning body fat, but—once again—the more muscle catabo-lism takes place. This is why I like only a loss of a pound or less per week. Muscle is being spared as much as possible and there are enough carbs in the diet to target workout energy levels and recovery.

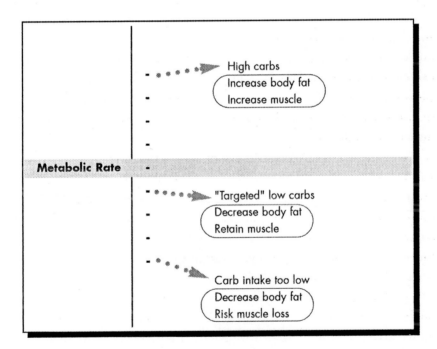

If protein levels are accurate and fat is minimal to moderate, carbs can fill the gap. My goal is for every client to diet on as high a carb intake as possible and still be achieving the goal. For a male ectomorph, this may be dieting on 350 grams per day, for an endomorph it may be 150 per day, but it's a relative phenomenon. The different metabolic rates and different body types dictate different food levels. Rat studies show tremendous differences in the liver's use of protein for energy based on carbohydrate intake. Low levels of carbs will allow non-contractile protein in the muscle and the liver to be used as energy, and lower levels of carb intake will start the process of using contractile protein from muscle tissue. Is there anything else on the planet that can cause a bodybuilder depression faster than that?! I mean, take my dog, take my girlfriend, but don't take an ounce of my muscle!!

Cycling is one method of walking this fine line. You can only go so long in carb depletion before you not only risk higher muscle loss, but you'll also be more prone to binge. It never fails to happen. When you go too low for too long with carb depletion, you'll hit the wall and go way overboard. I've heard all the stories; bags of Oreos, boxes of cereal, and enough candy to short-circuit your pancreas. If you have to diet on a lower-carb regimen, you have to plan a moderate increase every three to five days so that you can stay on track and do your best to prevent muscle loss.

Targeting your carbs is also essential. Prioritize your carbs so that you have them when they will help you preserve muscle the most. The most important time is your meal before your workout, then your post-workout meal, then breakfast, and spread the rest out evenly. If you're unlucky enough to be in a cycle where you're just not getting much, you should still prioritize them in this manner. If you only have enough for one meal, then have them before your workout, etc. This will provide glucose for energy so you'll use less muscle for energy while training, have more energy to lift heavier so you stimulate muscle growth/retention, and you'll whine less to your training partner about shrinkage.

All things considered, you'll have all the tools you need to maintain the most muscle possible while dieting.

1) Plan your offseason and precontest so you don't have to lose fat too quickly.

2) Set protein levels high enough but not excessively.

3) Set fat levels at no higher than 20% of total calories.

4) Set carb levels as high as possible while still staying on pace with weight loss.

5) Target your carbs to support muscle retention.

6) Cycle carbs if a prolonged low-carb run is necessary.

The Last Few Pounds

If it's difficult for you to lose the final few pounds, you're in good company. Many people have genes that let them get as lean as possible just by sticking to reasonable nutrition. Others among us end up eating less and doing more cardio as our body fat gets lower, and we still can't get that "thin-skinned" look.

I often utilize two variations of dieting for short periods of time with people that struggle with achieving the "shredded" physique. My version of a ketogenic diet is a bit subtler and a great deal healthier than the conventional plan. For a female, 50 grams of total carbs (almost all fiber) and for a male, 100 grams, should be the lowest you go. (Well, if you're up against time, you may go lower, but it gets tough!) Keep your protein intake the same as normal. The lack of carbs will encourage your body to convert excess protein to glucose, minimizing the effects of the lower carbs if you let your protein migrate upward. Keep your fat intake the same as well, and continue with healthy unsaturated fats. Within two-to-four days, you will severely deplete stored glycogen levels, increasing the rate of body fat breakdown for energy. You can go only so long, however, before you start losing muscle and decreasing your metabolism. Instead of wildly recarbing for two days out of every five (as is often suggested), you need only consume one large carbohydrate meal every three-to-six days, in addition to your normal daily intake. In other words, on every fourth day of consuming 100 grams of carbs, I would have one extra meal of 50 grams, making my daily total 150 grams for that fourth day. This three-day time span will keep you from having severe cravings, but if you can make it an additional day or two on the lower carbs, you'll lose fat faster. If you binge, however, you've blown the results and probably set yourself back to a net-zero for the week. This is extreme dieting, and the benefit is extreme body fat loss. The cost, however, is being tired, grouchy, and hungry, and you must have the mental discipline to endure what your body doesn't want to endure. If you try my version, or any other version, of the ketogenic diet and find yourself repeatedly failing or bingeing, give it up. You would be better off with slower but consistent results than with frustrating yo-yo dieting.

My second variation keeps carbs and fat the same as the first version, but instead of reloading with carbs, it uses extra protein to minimize hunger. Some people are so insulin-sensitive that a little increase in carbs leads to a wild binge. Protein digests slower, gives no opportunity for blood sugar spiking, and can effectively keep most people on a low-carb diet without too much suffering. Recall, however, that excess protein can be turned into glucose. Too much too often and you will counter the effects of the low-carb consumption and end up nowhere.

Either of these ketogenic versions should be used for no longer than four weeks before switching to "normal" weight loss nutrient totals for a couple of weeks. Cycling like this can be effective, or you can simply throw in a ketogenic cycle every once in awhile.

Metabolic Transformation in Action

"I was determined to be a winner in the INBF. While on vacation in April of 2002, I was working out in a gym in Cape Cod when I noticed a "ripped" woman. I knew she had to be a competitive bodybuilder so I approached her and she told me she owed all of her success to a body-builder/nutritionist, Dr. Joe Klemczewski. I contacted Joe and so began our road to my competition in June of that same year. I was willing to do whatever it took to win. I had dieted for competition on my own in 2001 and came in second place. I was told what I had to do to be a champ and I knew Joe would be my edge. He gave me exact details nutritionally and we communicated constantly; any time I needed Joe, he was there.

My biggest concern was dropping all the weight while keeping my muscle. I had gained fifty pounds in the offseason and had a long way to go.

The months that followed weren't always easy but I was determined to finish no matter what. Joe was with me every step of the way. When peak week arrived I was at 3.5% body fat and my weight was down to 180. I had lost fifty pounds of fat while retaining ALL of my muscle mass. During peak week it all came together. More vascularity and definition was present every day. Even on contest day, hour-by-hour I was getting fuller and harder. I won my first open division and immediately called Joe; I was so grateful for his help. It didn't stop there as I entered another show two months later. I was even sharper and won my open division and the overall title. I owe it all to Joe and with his help, this year I will be a professional bodybuilder! Thank you, Joe, I couldn't have done it without you."

Nick Montalbano, INBF Bodybuilder

Create Habits

Variety is important for being flexible, but habits are just as important. Creating good habits often gives us the structure we need to rely on. I know some very successful bodybuilders that eat the same meals at the same times every day without exception during a pre-contest phase.

Boring? Yes. But you can't ask for a more predictable, controllable outcome. The point is creating a pattern of meals, foods, and even treats that create the best results for you. I have developed several dieting habits, such as saving some of my carbs for air-popped popcorn to munch on in the evenings when I'm hungry. I have even done things as weird as putting just a half of a teaspoon of oats in a huge bowl of water, cooking it, adding cinnamon and—yum, yum—it's oatmeal-flavored water! When you're done laughing or throwing up, try it; you can get pretty filled up for only 10 grams of carbs with a couple bowls of this! If you think that's bad, I know a guy who will chew up a candy bar and spit it out one bite at a time without swallowing any of it! (Not recommended, by the way!)

Whatever good habits you can develop; use them for as long as you can. More examples: If you get hungry before it's time to eat, drink two glasses of water and get away from the kitchen—stay busy. Brush your teeth right after you eat so you're not tempted to go back for more. Drink flavored tea sweetened with a non-calorie sweetener like Stevia between meals. Eat more fibrous carbs like vegetables at meals to increase the amount of food volume that you can eat (10 cups of broccoli has the same carb content as 1 cup of rice). Chew your food *slowly*. Take small bites. Drink a gallon of water a day. Get enough sleep so you don't confuse fatigue with hunger/weakness.

Misery Loves Company

Find a friend or group of people that are pursuing the same goals. The motivation, accountability, and group learning can be tremendous. I often have clients that get to know each other and end up creating invaluable mini-support groups. I personally find it easier when I have someone right beside me each step of the way, striving toward the same goal.

Supplementation

Among hundreds of worthless supplements on health food store shelves, there are a few high-quality, safe, researched, and effective ones to chose from. There is plenty of material written on the following supplements, so I will simply tell you what I use and let you diligently look up the effects to decide which ones you may want to try. I personally use and often recommend some of the following supplements. True to my approach of dieting, I think muscle sparing should be a primary concern. Protein supplements are a key part of the diet just to make sure protein can be consumed in the amounts and at the rate of frequency required. L-glutamine is a "muscle feeding" amino acid that I used and recommended long before its re-popularization recently. It's inexpensive and a very capable companion to training and dieting. When in the hardest part of dieting, I also like branch chain amino acids (BCAAs) to combat catabolism. Ephedrine and caffeine stacks may soon be outlawed but have long been good appetite suppressants and energy boosters. The true fat-burning effects of ephedrine would require significant doses above what most people would be comfortable using, and certainly higher than I would ever recommend. If you use ephedrine, use it only for short durations—please study warnings and contraindications on labels. CLA is an essential fatty acid that has received some attention based on one study and shows promise. Whether there are significant fat-burning effects is still in question, but it is at least a good source of essential fatty acids. L-carnitine has long been a proven worthwhile amino acid for weight loss. Creatine, of course, is the most popular and most studied supplement in muscle-building history. It certainly does what it says for cellular hydration and anaerobic strength and power. But its effects are basically limited to the duration of usage. It's a "nutritional" supplement that our body produces and is available in protein sources. I recommend situational usage and, like most experts, to cycle off of it every few months if you do use it. Don't use any supplements you haven't fully researched or don't understand. Never use supplements in a way other than the way recommended by the manufacturer or distributor (as printed on the label).

Peak Week

I could fill a book with the quotes I hear at contests from competitors that placed second-through-last place in their classes. There are many versions, but just one quote. To paraphrase: "I screwed up my peak." It's usually sandwiched in a paragraph that includes phrases like carb loading, sodium manipulation, and water depletion, and it always comes right before the line, "I tried something new this time." I'm talking about legitimate peaking screw-ups, of which there are many. The one thing I want to eliminate from your mind at the beginning of this section is to blame your body fat percentage on peaking. Some people start peak week at 14 percent body fat and think that by doing one neat, new little trick that they read about, they'll wake up Saturday morning looking like Frank Zane. You've seen them. The ones at 8 percent body fat that say, "Yeah, I was just holding a little water today." This section isn't for them. This is for people that know how to dial in on contest shape and now want to know exactly what to do in order to wake up Saturday morning and shout, "Eureka! I did it!! I finally nailed my peak!!"

First of all, let's begin with how you should plan to enter peak week. If you still have to be concerned with losing "the last couple pounds" in the week before the show, you won't be able to peak properly. Peak week should be thought of as recovering slightly, being fresh, and making sure the muscles are full and hard, yet visible because of proper sub-cutaneous water elimination. Fat elimination should be over before this last week.

The next thing I want to erase from your thought process is the myth that you have to make extreme changes to manipulate your body into looking good on contest day. You've no doubt experimented with massive sodium loading and depletion, varying carb loading schemes, and endless water depletion schedules to try to be your biggest, hardest, and driest all at once. You also have probably experienced the shock of looking at a flat, shriveled up, smooth physique (with it's mouth gaping open in terror) in the mirror six hours before prejudging. DO NOT PLAN ON DOING ANYTHING DRASTIC DURING PEAK WEEK!!

Your body is constantly being monitored by your brain via thousands of chemoreceptors that are sending feedback on millions of chemical reactions happening in your body. It's how your brain manages to balance the chemical necessities of life. This vast neuro-hormonal-chemical network is brutally dynamic and always in flux. I'm not smart enough to predict and override these millions of reactions in my body to create an unnatural super-compensation effect exactly at prejudging and then maintain it all day. Neither are you. What we *can* do is understand the cycles that our body goes through in directing water into muscles or outside of the muscle cells, the way our body stores carbohydrates, and how to gently massage these cycles so that we ride the right wave into the right day and (predictably) peak perfectly and naturally instead of trying to force a freaky, extreme response. That is a gamble you'll lose 9 times out of 10.

When I peak a bodybuilder, I control protein, carbs, fat, sodium, water, and training. We start seven days from the show and I provide a chart that tells the athlete exactly what to do in what amounts on each day of the entire week. I use these variables to control the normal cycles of water and glycogen flow in and out of the muscle tissue. We start out the week in a certain pattern and then each day the variables change in a subtle way to be able to predict and control peaking. Obviously, every bodybuilder is different when it comes to the amounts of each variable. Some people have unbelievably fast metabolisms and some people are very carb-sensitive—two extreme differences that dictate different amounts of each nutrient variable and a slightly different schedule. But the actual flows and cycles are still very similar. It is important to know and understand what to expect on each day so you know how to adjust. For this reason, even my "online" clients around the country have daily communication with me during peak week. I want to go through each of these variables and give you some physiological insight as to why peaking is so elusive.

Carbing-up is the great myth of 250-pound steroid using bodybuilders that consume huge amounts of food anyway and then take prescription diuretics to eliminate their steroid bloat. If your body isn't a frenzied eighth grade science experiment, let's stick with normal physiology. Even the hardest, leanest bodies cannot metabolize and shuttle glucose into muscle cells at a maximum rate without having some extracellular spill-over. Read that sentence again. You cannot deplete carbs and then supercompensate and expect all of the glucose and water to end up in the muscle. You'll certainly fill out, but you'll also smooth out. Some a little, and some a great deal. Yes, a lot of carbs will go into the muscle, but a little or a lot will end up outside the muscle cells with a lot of water, which makes you smooth. Next time you're dieting and you're fairly lean, log some comments every day in a journal. "Woke up pretty lean. Very smooth—must have been the sodium in the chips. Very vascular. Hard as a freak'n rock!!" Just write down comments on how you look in the morning. I guarantee that you'll consistently be your hardest after a couple of low-carb, high-water intake days. You may not be your biggest because the carbs aren't as high, but the lack of extraneous carbs and water under the skin makes you very tight, and you appear much bigger. Who wins the show: the big soft guy or the bone-dry striated competitor? My method of carbing up my clients catches the wave of glucose and water entering the muscle on the way up, but not at the expense of smoothing out on the rebound effect of over-carbing.

My general carb cycle for peak week is to start at the highest point on the weekend before. I start at a slightly above "normal" level on Saturday and Sunday, and schedule no training. I want this weekend to be a recovery time, complete with a refilling of glycogen. After training starts again on Monday, I slowly drop carbs each day. It's a subtle drop, not a severe depletion. The training each day, Monday through

Wednesday, with the slight drop will create a sufficient carb deficit without total depletion. Depending on the client's metabolism, I keep the carbs coming down and keep the water very high all the way through Friday. For a very high metabolism bodybuilder, I'm not going as low on the carbs during the week, and I may start re-carbing on Friday. For carb-sensitive clients, it's very important to wait until Saturday to reload. By waiting until later in the week to carb up, you eliminate the chance of glycogen and water spillover. Your body can metabolize glucose very quickly, and you don't have to start three days ahead of time, especially if you haven't completely bottomed out due to severe carb depletion. There are also some issues with the type of carbs you use to reload. There are some that create more subcutaneous swelling due to being food allergens. It's important to know which are the most common and how they affect you.

Water is just as misunderstood as carbs. The traditional carb and water theories have people sometimes drop their water days before the show. Nothing will flatten and smooth you out faster! You have to maintain a high water intake because your muscle tissue is around 75 percent water. No water, no hardness—just flat, squishy muscle tissue. The reason people typically start dropping water is because they've over-carbed so much that they're already spilling glycogen and water under the skin and think, "Oh, my gosh!! I've got to get rid of this water!!" With the carb reload going as I described, you won't have that problem; you'll actually get harder and harder throughout the week. KEEP THE WATER INTAKE UP AND LET IT FOLLOW THE CARBS INTO THE MUSCLE!! IF YOU'RE NOT OVER-CARBED, THE REST OF THE WATER WILL BE ELIMI-NATED!!

Sodium also has to be tracked. Start with a moderate amount of sodium, up to two grams for females and up to three to four grams for males, at the beginning of the week, and on Friday, start dropping it slightly but don't eliminate it completely. If you do, you'll force water out of the muscle cell, you'll look flat and smooth, and you'll cramp like there's no tomorrow. You need approximately two times more sodium than potassium for your muscles to contract normally. Again, don't let the myths from the pharmaceutically dominated side of our sport lure you into doing things that aren't physiologically correct. If you sodium load and/or deplete in a big way, you're gambling with extreme chemical rebound effects that you can't possibly time. If you're lucky enough to stumble into a good effect, it will be short-lived because you're on a pendulum swing that your body will adjust to, and you'll look absolutely lousy in a very short time.

I also use specific tricks regarding fat intake, and schedule very specific contest day meal strategies for the individual needs and characteristics of my clients. As I get to know their metabolic rates throughout the dieting process, I'm already planning their peaks, and everyone's a little different. These general guidelines, however, will hopefully dispel some common mistakes and put you on a path to learning your body type and peaking perfectly every time!

Fluid Dynamics in Detail

While you drift in and out of sleep, your routine runs through your mind, your pulse races, and you wonder if "it will work." You are awake long before the alarm sounds, but you are afraid to look. Maybe just a little more sleep. Finally, you amble to the hotel bathroom, turn on the light, and slowly lift your shirt to reveal your abs. Will your skin be dry? Will deep crevices and vascularity be visible (as they were on so many days in the last two weeks)? Or...will you look soft...like last time?

There are countless locker room experts to guide you through the last week of your contest preparation. They competed a decade ago in the County Novice Mr. Nobody, have their PhD from Flex Magazine, and their advice is free. You listened. It sounded logical at the time because they were so confident. If my psychic powers are tuned correctly and Jupiter is in the right position, I bet I can get close to your formula. Carb deplete Sunday through Tuesday, drink tons of water, maybe sodium load a little, carb load starting Wednesday, start cutting water Thursday (Friday virtually none), eliminate sodium for two or three days prior to Saturday, start taking 99 mg of potassium every two hours, and use a magic cocktail of glycerol, creatine, and sugar (toss in a little wine if you're on the British team), and finish it all up with an over-the-counter dandelion root-based diuretic to supercharge your vascularity. By the way, if you ever get tired of bodybuilding, pharmaceutical companies pay volunteers to test new therapies that are far less complicated—you may want to apply.

Metabolic Transformation in Action

"Before Dr. Joe began helping me with nutrition, training, and "peak week," I gathered my information from many different sources. I read magazine articles, talked to fellow competitors, and even took advice from people who had never competed! It was a guessing game for me. I used various techniques just hoping they would work. Unfortunately I found out that the information available to bodybuilders varies greatly and is often based on product sales or misguided athletes. It was extremely difficult to know what advice to follow and what might work the best, especially for my body and contest goals.

Dr. Joe provided me with individualized strategies to help me come in at my best. His scientific approach helped me target in on specific goals. Working with Joe has been a true learning experience. Because of his help, I now know how to manipulate my training and diet to be perfectly dialed in on contest day.

Most importantly, Joe's scientific approach to contest training and dieting is healthier and more sensible than many of the methods I had used in the past. Dr. Joe's advice is easier to follow and produces better results. I've learned more about contest nutrition from him than anywhere else. He knows his stuff!"

photo by Sandra Lynch

Kent Julius, WNBF Mr. International

I know I'm being cruel. How can I joke about this when you're standing in front of the mirror shocked by how you could follow the protocol so perfectly yet you're flatter and softer than you were last Saturday? I hate to tell you, but it will get worse. After the disappointment of not being able to recover your form all day, you'll wake up tomorrow full, hard, and vascular. Sunday, that is…just like last year. Why is it so hard to time a peak? Turn off the TV, you're going to want to concentrate on this section.

Water balance in your body is incredibly complex. The end goal of a bodybuilder on contest day is to look "hard." Body fat must be gone, that's a given, but even with the leanest physique you can present, the shredded/dry look comes from having a minimal amount of water under your skin. Really, what this means is interstitial plasma, which can be thought of as any fluid outside the cells in your body. There are several processes that affect cellular fluid dynamics. We have to start with the big picture.

Water makes up 50-60 percent of your body and up to 75 percent of your muscle tissue. If you're 2 percent dehydrated, it will negatively affect your muscle tissue and athletic ability. If you're 5 percent dehydrated you'll cramp, and if you're 7-10 percent dehydrated you'll hallucinate and risk death. Think back to when you were drinking a gallon and a half of water a day. You were full, hard, and vascular. Why? You had enough water in your body. The morning of the show you were flat as a pancake, soft as a marshmallow, and every muscle in your body shook and cramped on stage. Why? You were dehydrated. When you see pictures of top WNBF pros that are clients of mine, you can trust that they didn't cut water one bit.

Why weren't they waterlogged and soft? The water was in their muscle tissue making them full and hard, while interstitial water was at a minimum. Keeping water intake normal gives you the opportunity to be full, but being hard depends on what we do to channel it into the muscle. This is where the sodium/potassium comes in. Sodium is the major extracellular fluid cation, and potassium is the major intracellular fluid cation. Aha!! Professor Novice Mr. Nobody was right in having me cut sodium and increase potassium! Nope. Misapplied science. Normal physiology maintains 55-65 percent of our fluid intracellularly anyway. If we are in normal condition, we have more fluid inside than outside our cells. It's when we screw something up that this percentage heads in the other direction and fluid is diverted outside the cell. Fluid dynamics is controlled with incredible precision via our kidneys. Though you hear the phrase "you have to trick your body" every time you get a locker room lesson on peaking, trust me: there is no tricking your body. It's much faster than you are and much more sophisticated than you could ever hope to account for. Every time you do something extreme trying to cause an extreme reaction, you'll get one. Two problems are: first, it may not be the one you wanted, and second, if it is, it will be very short-lived because the extreme reaction will be quickly countered in the other direction just as severely until the "pendulum" that you violently swung slows back down. Take a serious look at what happened to your body during the fictitious example I gave. You went from hard and full, to harder, then a little smaller, then huge, then huge and soft, then soft and flat on the morning of the show, then huge and vascular on Sunday, and finally as soft and squishy as can be for a couple days after that. That's the kind of instability you get when you start trying to "trick" your body.

Yes, sodium and potassium are key ions that regulate cellular fluid dynamics, but you can't create extreme environments and expect to time them. You can subtly influence them, but keep in mind this phrase: "water follows solutes." Water is attracted to and will follow the ions as they travel across the cell membranes. We want plasma to be attracted to the inside of the cell, but it won't happen by just increasing potassium. The goal should be to simply maintain the "normal," stable environment that would have 55-65 percent of the fluid there anyway. Just as big a factor, however, is sodium and its role in blood volume. Deficiencies in sodium will lead to a drop in blood pressure, which means plasma has been pushed out of the vascular system.

If it's not in your blood vessels, it's around them interstitially, which means subcutaneously. That, of course, means SMOOTH!! This will then start a chain reaction that will take days to remedy. When sodium is dropped from the diet, your kidneys will be influenced immediately by the hormone Aldosterone to conserve sodium from being excreted, and remember: water follows solutes. If sodium is being reabsorbed, then water will be as well. You retain water and, with lower blood pressure, it's all under your skin instead of in your vascular system.

Take a look at this study:

NORMAL DIET	LOW SODIUM:		
	1 day	2 days	6 days
Urinary Sodium 217 (mmol/day)	105	59	9.9
Aldosterone 10.4 (ng/100 ml)	11.7	22.5	37
Serum Sodium 139 (mmol)	139	139	138

Within one day of dropping dietary sodium, excreted sodium is cut in half and continues to decline as more Aldosterone is produced. BUT, look at blood levels of sodium: they're conserved perfectly!! YOU CAN'T TRICK YOUR BODY!! All you did by cutting sodium was screw up the osmolarity of the cell membranes, and you won't know where the water is going to go. If you keep your water intake and sodium intake normal, your cellular fluid dynamics will stay normal. So, you ask, "What's normal?" The RDA for sodium is a range of .5-2.4 grams per day but other sources recommend up to 3.3 grams per day. The RDA for potassium is 1.6-2.0 grams per day. One quick side note on potassium: excessive potassium will also stimulate Aldosterone. Don't add potassium in amounts that place it higher than sodium intake. Everyone, of course, is a little different, and this is precisely why I don't just "peak" clients. I have to spend more than a week working with them so I can make and observe changes in their bodies before I detail a perfect plan for them as individuals.

I know you may be disappointed to hear all this talk about "normal," so I want to give you a chance to manipulate a variable that WILL make a huge difference. Since I won't let you whack your sodium/potassium around, what other nutrient could possibly affect water balance in a very, very positive way??

Carbs. You already know that every gram of glycogen (stored glucose/carbohydrate) attracts water to it—2.7 grams of water, to be exact. Remember the "water follows solutes" thing? Glycogen is a solute, too. This is why you get so full and feel so huge when your carbs are high. Your water content is also high. We already established that when your water is low, you'll experience the opposite: flat, soft muscles. The real trick is to have enough carbs in your body to attract water in your muscle tissue to be full and hard, but you may have also heard the phrase "spilling over" in relation to carbs. This is a legitimate concern. The average adult can only store 375-475 grams of carbs in the body, about 325 of which would be in the muscle (90-110 grams in the liver and 15-20 as blood glucose). When you consume too many carbohydrates, which is likely with a traditional carb-up, the excessive glycogen ends up in the interstitial fluids, the water follows, and now there's another reason for the water under your skin. How you carb up, how much you carb up with, and the foods you use are all factors in making sure the glucose is in the muscle, not outside. Combine this with water intake, sodium/potassium intake, and even your training, and you have the full picture of how you will look on Saturday morning.

I know this is an incredibly complex section, but if you read it, make notes, and sort it out, you'll see that peaking can be consistent and predictable, not a gamble. I'll let you go back through this material to isolate the details, but I hope I have impressed upon you that dropping water, eliminating sodium, increasing potassium, and carbing up hard are not only physiologically contrary to your goals, they are probably sabotaging your contest days! Try doing things in concert with your body instead of trying to trick it, and practice these things several times before contest day!

Invest in Proper Education

It would be embarrassing to me if I added up all the money I've ever wasted trying to do something cheap, or all the time I've wasted trying to cut corners, only to have to "do it right" the second time around. You have probably shaken your head in bewilderment as you've watched the same people make the same mistakes at the gym and wonder why they never progress. A small investment in a good personal trainer can lead to a cumulative level of progress that is otherwise unattainable. Similarly, an expert in nutrition can lead you to personal knowledge that you may never otherwise obtain. Clients that become members of our facility and stay in communication with our staff end up becoming very competent very quickly. Someone that comes in only once would have a great disadvantage. For this reason alone, I have created the "On-line" program to compliment this book. Inexperienced bodybuilders or physique extremists trying to get lean for the first time or trying for their all-time best condition often need day-to-day help. Pushing past metabolic set points requires walking a fine line between maximum fat loss, keeping the metabolic rate high, and maintaining muscle mass. Nutrient cycling and alternating phases of varying cardio are complicated but very important. Clients such as these are in contact with me at least every other day, and get great results. Not only do they achieve their immediate goals, but the investment provides detailed documentation for them to refer back to. Whether this book is the final piece of your metabolic puzzle, or just your starting point, I pray it serves you well.

BIBLIOGRAPHY

Abbasi, F., et al. 2000. "High carbohydrate diets, triglyceride rich lipo-proteins, and coronary heart disease risk." *American Journal of Cardiology* 85:45-48.

Acheson, K. J., et al. 1984. "Nutritional influences on lipogenesis and thermogenesis after a carbohydrate meal." *American Journal of Physiology* 246:E62-E70.

Agus, M. S. D., et al. 2000. "Dietary composition and physiologic adaptations to energy restriction." *American Journal of Clinical Nutrition* 71:901-7.

Ascherio, A., and W. C. Willet. 1997. "Health effects of transfatty acids." *American Journal of Clinical Nutrition* 66:1006S-1010S.

Atkins, R.C. 2002. *Dr. Atkins' New Diet Revolution.* Avon, New York, NY.

Baba, N. H., et al. 1999. "High protein versus high carbohydrate hypoenergetic diet for the treatment of obese hyperinsulinemic subjects." *International Journal of Obesity* 11:1202-1206.

Brand-Miller, J. C. et al. 2002. "Glycemic index and obesity." *American Journal of Clinical Nutrition* 76:281S-285S.

Brand-Miller, J., et al. 2003. *The New Glucose Revolution.* Marlowe and Company, New York, NY.

Brody, Tom. 1999. *Nutritional Biochemistry,* Second ed. Academic Press, San Diego, CA.

Campfield, L., F. Smith, and P. Burn. 1998. "Strategies and potential molecular targets for obesity treatment." *Science* 280:1383-1387.

Carlola, R., J. P. Harley, and C. R. Noback. 1990. *Human Anatomy and Physiology.* McGraw-Hill, New York, NY.

Chinachoti, P. 1995. "Carbohydrates: Functionality in foods." *American Journal of Clinical Nutrition* 61:922S-929S.

Crapo, P. A. 1985. "Simple versus complex carbohydrate use in the diabetic diet." *Annual Review of Nutrition* 5:95-114.

Daly, M. E. et al. 1997. "Dietary carbohydrate and insulin sensitivity: A review of the evidence and clinical implications." *American Journal of Clinical Nutrition* 66:1072-1085.

Depres, J-P., et al. 1996. "Hyperinsulinemia as an independent risk factor for ischemic heart disease." *New England Journal of Medicine* 334:952-957.

Dune, L. J. 1990. *Nutrition Almanac,* 3rd ed. McGraw-Hill, New York, NY.

Eades, M. R. and M. D. Eades. 1996. *Protein Power.* Bantam Books, New York, NY.

Ely, D. L. 1997. "Overview of dietary sodium effects on and interactions with cardiovascular and neuroendocrine functions." *American Journal of Clinical Nutrition* 65:594S-605S.

Erikson, R. H. and Y. S. Kim. 1990. "Digestion and absorption of dietary protein." *Annual Review of Medicine* 41:133-139.

Felig, P., et al. 1970. "Amino acid metabolism in the regulation of gluconeogenesis in man." *American Journal of Clinical Nutrition* 23:986-992.

Felig, P., J. D. Baxter, and L. A. Frohman. 1995. *Endocrinology and Metabolism*, 3rd ed. McGraw_Hill, New York, NY.

Figlewicz, D. P., et al. 1996. "Endocrine regulation of food intake and body weight." *Journal of Laboratory and Clinical Medicine* 127:328-332.

Fisler, J. S., et al. 1982. "Nitrogen economy during very low calorie reducing diets." *American Journal of Clinical Nutrition* 35:471-486.

Ford, E. S., and S. Liu. 2001. "Glycemic index and serum high-density-lipoprotein cholesterol concentration among US adults." *Archives of Internal Medicine* 161:572-48.

Fordslund, A. H., et al. 1999. "Effect of protein intake and physical activity on twenty-four hour pattern and rate of micronutrient utilization." *American Physiology Society* E964-E976.

Foster-Powell, K., J. C. Brand-Miller, S. H. A. Holt. 2002. "International table of glycemic index and glycemic load values: 2002." *American Journal of Clinical Nutrition* 76:5-56.

Friedman, H. I. And B. Nylund. 1980. "Intestinal fat digestion, absorption, and transport." *American Journal of Clinical Nutrition* 33:1108-1139.

Frost, G. and A. Dornhorst. 2000. "The relevance of the glycemic index to our understanding of dietary carbohydrates." *Diabetic Medicine* 17:336-45

Fushiki, T., et al. 1989. "Changes in glucose transporters in muscle in response to glucose." *American Journal of Physiology* 256:E580-E587.

Golay, A., et al. 1996. "Weight loss with low or high carbohydrate diet?" *International Journal of Obesity and Related Metabolic Disorders* 20:1067-1072.

Gottfried, S. S. 1993. *Biology Today.* Mosby, St. Louis, MO.

Groff, J. L. and S. S. Gropper. 2000. *Advanced Nutrition and Human Metabolism.* Wadsworth Thomson Learning, Stamford, CT.

Holloszy, J. and W. Kohrt. 1996. "Regulation of carbohydrate and fat metabolism during and after exercise." *Annual Review of Nutrition* 16:121-138.

Holman, R. T. 1988. "George O. Burr and the discovery of essential fatty acids." *Journal of Nutrition* 118:535-540.

Hudgins, L., et al. 2000. "Relationship between carbohydrate induced hypertriglyceridemia and fatty acid synthesis in lean and obese subjects." *Journal of Lipid Research* 41:595-604.

Leaf, A. and P. C. Weber. 1988. "Cardiovascular effects of n-3 fatty acids." *New England Journal of Medicine* 318:549-557.

Leeds, A. R. 2002. "Glycemic index and heart disease." *American Journal of Clinical Nutrition* 76:286S-289S.

Leibel, R. L., M. Rosenbaum, and J. Hirsch. 1995. "Changes in energy expenditure resulting from altered body weight." *New England Journal of Medicine* 332:621-628.

Leibowitz, S. F. 1992. "Neurochemical-neuroendocrine systems in the brain controlling macronutrient intake and metabolism." *Trends in Neuroscience* 15:491-497.

Jacobson, M. F. and J. Hurley. 2002. *Restaurant Confidential.* Workman Publishing, New York, NY.

McArdle, W. D., F. I. Katch, and V. L. Katch. 1991. *Exercise Physiology: Energy, Nutrition, and Human Performance,* Third ed. Lea and Febiger, Malvern, PA.

Millward, D.J. 1998. "Metabolic demands for amino acids and the human dietary requirement." *Journal of Nutrition* 2563S-2576S.

Morris, K., et al. 1999. "Glycemic index, cardiovascular disease, and obesity." *Nutrition Reviews* 57:273-276.

Murray, M. T. and J. Beutler. 1996. *Understanding Fats and Oils.* Progressive Health Publishing, Encinitas, CA.

Nelson, J. K., et al. 1994. *Mayo Clinic Diet Manual: A Handbook of Nutrition Practices,* Seventh ed. Mosby, St. Louis, MO.

Netzer, C.T. 2003. *The Complete Book of Food Counts.* Dell Publishing, New York, NY.

Nicholl, C. G., J. M. Polak, and S. R. Bloom. 1985. "The hormonal regulation of food intake, digestion, and absorption." *Annual Review of Nutrition* 5:213-239.

Nobels, F., et al. 1989. "Weight reduction with a high protein, low carbohydrate, caloric restricted diet: Effects on blood pressure, glucose, and insulin levels." *Netherlands Journal of Medicine* 35:295-302.

Pieke., B., et al. 2000. "Treatment of hypertriglyceridemia by two diets rich either in unsaturated fatty acids or in carbohydrates: Effects on lipoprotein subclasses, lipolytic enzymes, lipid transfer proteins, insulin, and leptin. *International Journal of Obesity* 24:1286-1296.

Pilkis, S. J., et al. 1988. "Hormonal regulation of hepatic gluconeogenesis and glycolysis." *Annual Review of Biochemistry* 57:755-783.

Reed, W. D., et al. 1984. "The effects of insulin and glucagons on ketone-body turnover." *Biochemistry* 221:439-444.

Reeds, P.J. and T. W. Hutchens. 1994. "Protein requirements: From nitrogen balance to functional impact." *Journal of Nutrition* 1754S-1963-S.

Richter, E. A., T. Ploug, and H. Galbo. 1985. "Increased muscle glucose uptake after exercise." *Diabetes* 34:1041-1048.

Scriver, C. R., et al. 1985. "Normal plasma amino acid values in adults: The influence of some common physiological variables." *Metabolism* 34:868-873.

Sears, B. and B. Lawren. 1995. *Enter the Zone.* Harper Collins, New York, NY.

Souba, W. W., R. J. Smith, and D. W. Wilmore. 1985. "Glutamine Metabolism by the intestinal tract." *Journal of Parenteral Enteral Nutrition* 9:608-617.

Thorne, A. and J. Wahren. 1989. "Diet-induced thermogenesis in well-trained subjects." *Clinical Physiology* 0:295-305.

Traxinger, R. R. and S. Marshall. 1989. "Role of amino acids in modulating glucose-induced desensitization of the glucose transport system." *Journal of Biological Chemistry* 264:20910-20916.

Westphal, S. A., M. C. Gannon, and F. Q. Nutrall. 1990. "Metabolic response to glucose ingested with various amounts of protein." *American Journal of Clinical Nutrition* 62:267-272.

Whitney, E. N. and S. R. Rolfes. 1996. *Understanding Nutrition,* Seventh ed. West Publishing Company, St. Paul, MN.

Woods, S. C., et al. 1998. "Signals that regulate food intake and energy homeostasis." *Science* 280:1378-1383.

Wolfe, B. M. 1995. "Potential role of raising dietary protein intake for reducing risk of atherosclerosis." *Canadian Journal of Cardiology* 11:127G-131G.

Yamada, T., et al. 1995. *Textbook of Gastroenterology,* Second ed. J.B. Lippincott Company, Philadelphia, PA.

Young, D. B., et al. 1984. "Effects of sodium intake on steady-state potassium excretion." *American Journal of Physiology* 246:F772-F778.

Young, V. R. and J. S. Marchini. 1990. "Mechanisms and nutritional significance of metabolic responses to altered intakes of protein and amino acids, with reference to nutritional adaptation in humans." *American Journal of Clinical Nutrition* 51:270-289.

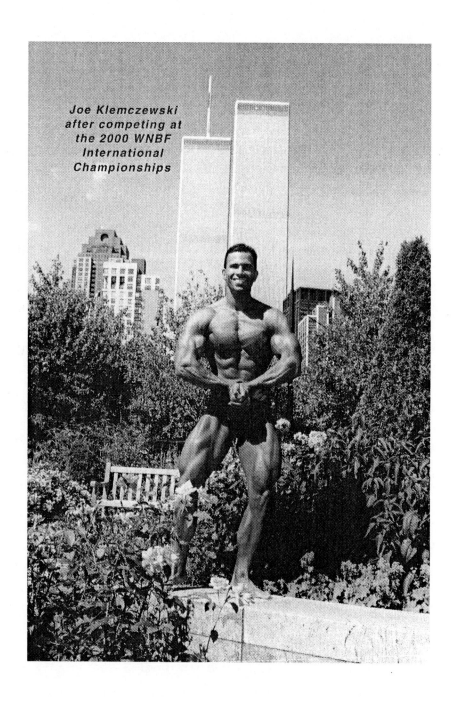

*Joe Klemczewski
after competing at
the 2000 WNBF
International
Championships*

ABOUT THE AUTHOR

Athletics led Dr. Klemczewski to weight training by the age of 13, and he competed in his first bodybuilding contest at the age of 20. By the age of 27, he won his pro card with the World Natural Bodybuilding Federation (WNBF).

Klemczewski received his Bachelor of Science degree in Physical Therapy from the Indiana University School of Medicine. While working as an orthopedic outpatient physical therapist, he continued his education by earning graduate degrees in health- and nutrition-related fields. Along the way, he also studied for and passed the renowned Certified Strength and Conditioning Specialist examination through the National Strength and Conditioning Association (NSCA).

Shortly after finishing his doctorate and winning his pro card, Dr. Joe developed a small, private gym complete with a nutritional program and physical therapy services. He expanded the facility with quality staff, and it has become a local and regional household name.

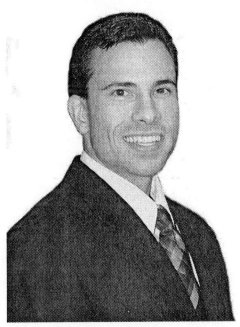

Almost four years ago, he founded Genetitec, Inc., a supplement company specializing in proprietary protein formulations. His research and product development changed the entire landscape of the supplement industry. Klemczewski's nutrition articles have been published in several magazines.

He has now turned his attention to his new company, Dr. Joe's Revolution—Center for Training and Nutrition, and his weekly radio show, Revolution with Dr. Joe: America's Permanent Weight Loss Expert. Most of Joe's time is now spent with nutritional program development for both local and national clients through his acclaimed online consulting program. Information can be found on his website at www.joesrevolution.com. He also conducts nationwide motivational and instructional workshops on various nutritional topics. Joe resides in Evansville, Indiana, with his wife Tracy and their four children.

For information, write to Genesis Health Systems, Inc., 915 Main Street, Suite 406, Evansville, IN 47708.

0-595-29268-2

Printed in the United States
44254LVS00005B/366